Sexy Birth

Dayna Martin

FREELIFE PRESS

Sexy Birth

Copyright © 2012 Dayna Martin

www.DaynaMartin.com

Cover and back photos by Jay Philbrick, www.philbrickphoto.com
Editing by Lynda Miles, blmiles@hotmail.com

Freelife Press Paperback edition 2012
www.freelifepress.com

Printed in the United States of America
First Printing, 2012

DEDICATION

This book is dedicated you, the reader. It is your birthright and my intention that by having a *Sexy Birth*, you will experience empowerment and joy beyond belief. It is also my hope that this will be the start of a relationship with your child based on love, connection and trust, rather than the cultural mindset of fear and control.

"If we hope to create a non-violent world where respect and kindness replace fear and hatred, we must begin with how we treat each other at the beginning of life. For that is where our deepest patterns are set. From these roots grow fear and alienation ~ or love and trust."

SUZANNE ARMS

TABLE OF CONTENTS

FOREPLAY

Finding out you are pregnant is one of the most pivotal times in a woman's life. Your entire future rolls out in front of you, as you are confronted with decisions and choices you have never thought about before. You come to a place in your life where taking full responsibility for yourself and another life, is on your shoulders. Many women aren't ready for this aspect of womanhood; this can lead to a birth experience that she regrets for the rest of her life.

Birth can be traumatic or it can be empowering; it can be full of fear or it can be full of love and trust. What she creates for herself and her baby is entirely the woman's responsibility.

The thoughts she has during pregnancy are the leading factors in what she creates as her own life experience. Her thoughts and feelings surrounding birth are a driving force in the creation of the baby itself. As she embarks on the rite of passage that is *birth*, her thoughts and feelings are also a driving force in her own evolution as woman.

How a baby enters this world has a profound impact on that human being and his mother for the rest of their lives. When a baby is born in love, joy and trust, that foundation is the place from which everything else grows for both of them–for the rest of their lives.

Being responsible for your birth means shifting from a cultural place of control, to a place of trust and inner knowing that *all is well* and as it should be. It is a space of acceptance for what is; then from that disposition of well-being, informed decisions can be made. A place of fear or worry isn't the best place to be when making decisions; but unfortunately, in our culture, fear is what fuels most decisions. It is no wonder that birth becomes something very scary for most women.

For most women, making decisions from a place of well-being is a very different way to handle the decisions surrounding birth. From the moment we are born, we are taught that we are not to be trusted, and that the world is a scary place where we have to prepare for worst-case scenarios. In my experience, when birth is handled like a crisis waiting to happen–crisis usually happens, in some way, shape or form. The Universe is very obedient in that way!

When you reside in the space of knowing all is well and tune into the unique needs of your body, pregnancy and birth can be profoundly different from the cultural norm! Trusting–not fearing the processes–brings forth a creation of an amazingly positive experience, and sets the stage for motherhood to be joyful, instinctual and fulfilling. The only way to truly connect with your baby is through trusting the process, because trusting means loving. You can't fully love with fear leading the emotional parade!

Birth is on a continuum of sexuality that stretches from conception, to labor, and, finally, the birth of your child itself. Birth doesn't have to be scary, a medical emergency, or something that you turn over to professionals to manage. You have everything within you to grow your baby and also to give birth. Your baby is, after all, a physical manifestation of love itself.

A *Sexy Birth* is a birth where trust and love are the predominant emotions guiding you through the entire process. Most women and professionals in our culture do not view birth in such a positive way; so much of it, they believe, is just by chance or luck. Nothing could be further from the truth!

By learning to focus your thoughts on what you want–having a joyful, healthy and positive birth experience–you are able to create just that! By taking full responsibility for what you read, whom you surround yourself with, and what kinds of thoughts you choose about labor and birth, you will have the birth of your dreams.

There is a big difference between being aware of options–in case of the slightest chance that a variation comes up during your labor and birth–and focusing on all that could go wrong. In our culture, people tend to think that over-preparing for the worst is the safest way to live: but science and nature are showing us, that by doing this, we are actually *creating* the worst-case scenarios.

It is really very simple, and once you realize this, you can see how this common approach to birth–and to life itself–has led so many people in a direction, opposite of the one they would like to be headed in.

Birth can only be positive when you have a positive outlook, and trust yourself and your body. Focusing on what is *likely* to happen, which is that all will go perfectly, is the safest and healthiest emotional place to be, during your pregnancy and birth.

By focusing on and thinking about worst-case scenarios, you make it more *likely* that they will happen. I cannot say this enough! You can be *aware* of slight variations that *may* come up, but for the best chance of birth going perfectly, you must *control your thoughts* and strive to feel good, both physically and emotionally. Focus all of your thoughts on what you *do* want, not what you don't want. Feeling good is the secret to having the healthiest, safest and most joyful birth possible.

Birth is safe, easy and profoundly transforming if you know what to be thinking, and what to be feeling during the experience. That is just what this book will help you accomplish: a joyful, confident mindset about birth, simply through learning how to feel good.

All you have to do to create this for yourself is to take the time to learn about this new birthing paradigm! This leading-edge perspective about pregnancy and birth will show you how powerful you really are, and how you can create your own reality and experiences in life. When you do this, you truly can have a powerful, positive and fabulous *Sexy Birth!*

Sexy Birth

1

JOURNEY TO MY SEXY BIRTH

I have given birth four times. After the birth of my firstborn son, Devin, my life was forever changed. We had just connected to the Internet and information was available in a way that I had never experienced before. I knew that I wanted a natural birth, and I began learning about this whole new world (one that I had previously thought was for "granola-types" and "hippies").

I never knew the benefits of bringing a child into this world, without drugs or intervention. The more research I did, the more certain I was that *going natural* was the way for me. I hired a midwife and began a relationship with her, built on trust and support.

My first time around, my labor was fast and powerful and I gave birth to a 9.6 lb. baby. It was the most incredible, life-changing moment in my life. I never knew that I could be the type of woman that I had been reading about, for the past nine months.

My dream came true, and I was so grateful for that moment when I reached down and felt his warm, wet head coming out of my body. It was all so surreal, that there was really a human inside of me all of that time during my pregnancy; and he was *mine*–my baby, my child, my son. It was the beginning of an entirely new identity and purpose for my life.

No one ever told me that birth could be joyful, life-changing or powerful. No one ever told me that it would give me confidence and heal my emotional pain from the past. In the instant of bringing forth life, I was reborn and had recreated myself.

Within moments of his birth, I knew that I had to share this incredible message of empowerment with other women, so that they could understand the significance of birth in their lives. I wanted others to know how essential it is to go through the natural process of labor and birth, in order to reach their full potential as women and to evolve to the next stage on their own life path. I had found my true calling.

After the birth of my son, the choices surrounding parenting itself became even more complex. The people in my life, who were the most loving and supportive, suddenly became the most opinionated and controlling. I was given unsolicited advice at every turn. When I held my son, I was warned not to hold him too much. When I nursed him, I was asked when I would wean him. When I shared that he slept next to me at night, family and friends gasped in fear and disbelief.

By bringing him forth into this world the way nature intended, my mothering instincts were strongly intact, so I was not swayed by the fear and opinions of others. When my husband, Joe, and I began making choices that were not in alignment with the cultural norm, we were met with rejection, shame and fear, from everyone around us. We were so alone, yet we were not alone. We had our little family and it was all that we truly needed.

During this time, I learned to love and trust myself in a new way. No one would tell me how to raise my child! I became a fiercely protective and confident mother. For the first time in my life, I didn't doubt myself or my choices. Others' fears and rejection actually gave me confidence, because I knew that we had to be strong to parent from the heart.

We realized that we would be walking our parenting path with little support, unless I actively sought it out. I joined groups online, with people who were all parenting in a similar way. These new online friends were all respecting their children in a way that I had never heard about before! I learned about,

"Attachment Parenting" and was able to place a label on how we were choosing to parent. I was introduced to a whole new world that resonated with my heart and instincts.

I bought a used baby sling, when my son was only a few weeks old. We sold the crib, bought a bigger bed and enjoyed nighttime parenting, as we proudly and confidentially shared a *family bed*.

Our identity as people shifted dramatically, but it felt so good and so right! Through birth and mothering in a way that felt right to me, I had grown to be a joyful and confident mother. I had evolved as a person and loved our path deeply. I had a zest for life and a passion for mothering, birthing and breastfeeding. A fire was lit and so was my passion for sharing how incredible parenting could be, when you listen to your instincts from a place of trust and not fear.

Soon, my life's goal was to help other mothers know this secret of joyful parenting: Women are strong, capable and powerful and when you listen to your heart, you can do things that you never had the confidence to do before. You can reinvent yourself and become the person that you were meant to be in life by tuning into your instincts–something that is trained out of most people very early in life in our authoritarian culture.

I began studying to be a childbirth educator, Doula and breastfeeding counselor. I could not get enough information about birth and parenting! It felt so good to learn everything I could about the alternative birthing and parenting culture! I loved pouring through books and websites, and anytime I had a spare moment, I was researching, growing and connecting with others who were on the same path.

I was in research mode for two years of my life and I lived and breathed my passion, both in practice and in my studies. Soon after I became a certified childbirth educator, Doula and La Leche League Leader, I had my first homebirth with my daughter, Dakota.

A homebirth isn't something that I considered when I was pregnant the first time. Until I entered this whole new paradigm of birth and parenting, I had never heard of anyone choosing to have their baby at home.

Joe was a little nervous when I first told him about my desire, so we met with the homebirth midwives. He felt much more at ease, once his questions and fears were respectfully addressed. He asked them about emergency situations, and all of the "what-ifs" that so many people bombard you with, when they first hear that you are making an alternative choice in birth.

The birth of Dakota was another rite of passage, because birthing at home brings a woman to a whole new understanding of how truly safe birth is. You feel so much more comfortable about birthing, in general, when you realize that all of the fears, surrounding homebirth, are the result of misinformation and lack of education.

Homebirth isn't just for "fringe" people, whom others view as weird or different. Homebirth is for the average, mainstream, everyday pregnant woman! It truly is, and when you begin researching it, you will see more and more that it is being accepted and even praised by the mainstream! Homebirth is for YOU, if you want it to be.

For as long as we can remember, we are raised to fear birth! On television and in movies, we see images of women screaming in agony, begging for drugs, while they curse their partners for "doing this to them." I am here to share that it is *all a lie and a perpetuation of keeping women in the victim role.*

When you understand your power, and release these old ingrained ideas about birth, you can step up and take the necessary responsibility to have the birth you want.

 None of the common ideas about birth hold true, when you take responsibility for your own experience. When you take the power into your own hands, you aren't even in the same category as women who have someone else manage their births.

It is in the management of birth, that the fear, pain and risks come into the picture, because only *you* know what you want and need, to feel confident and comfortable. When someone else controls the situation, it never goes the way you want it to, *ever*.

By the time I was planning my third birth with my second daughter, Ivy, I had already been a childbirth educator and Doula for several years. I had attended the births of other women and had witnessed birth, both in the way that nature intended and in situations where it was very medically managed.

There were some variations in birth, like posterior labors, that scared me very much. A posterior labor is when the baby is turned around, in the mother, so the baby's spine is against the mother's spine. It causes a lot of back pain during the labor and birth. Although I witnessed these women birthing naturally with this uncommon variation, it seemed very painful.

During my pregnancy with Ivy, I began doing exercises every day to *prevent* a posterior labor. I began researching how to *avoid* having a posterior birth. I even went to a hypnotist to address my obsessive fear. So much of my focus was on *preventing* a posterior. Well, can you guess what kind of labor I had, once I finally went into labor? You guessed it… she was *posterior*.

It was the most challenging labor and birth that I had ever experienced–or even witnessed. It was long and painful and it was exactly what had I feared for nine months. I was grateful she was born at home and that I did it, but the experience was traumatic for me. I pushed for six hours and finally had an almost eleven pound baby girl, who was born posterior.

How on earth did this happen after all I did to prevent it? Why did I experience exactly what I'd feared and focused on and prepared so much for?!

After working with women as a birth professional for over a decade, I have learned the reason why: **a woman attracts to birth whatever she gives most of her attention, energy and focus to-whether wanted or unwanted.**

Your dominant thoughts are *exactly* what you bring into your birth experience. I had never heard about this before, but once I understood it, I felt as though I learned the secret to not only a positive, joyful birth-but to life itself.

"This entire reality is your creation. Feel good about that. Feel grateful for the richness of your world. And then begin creating the reality you truly want by making decisions and holding intentions. Think about what you desire, and withdraw your thoughts from what you don't want. The most natural, easiest way to do this is to pay attention to your emotions.

Thinking about your desires feels good, and thinking about what you don't want makes you feel bad. When you notice yourself feeling bad, you've caught yourself thinking about something you don't want. Turn your focus back towards what you do want, and your emotional state will improve rapidly. As you do this repeatedly, you'll begin to see your physical reality shift too, first in subtle ways and then in bigger leaps. You suddenly see that everything that has happened to you in life is a result of your own creation through what you were thinking about and focusing on." Steve Pavlina

This powerful shift of taking full responsibility in my life, led me to my final and most profound birthing experience: *the birth of my son, Orion*. During my pregnancy with Orion, I did something I hadn't done with the other three pregnancies. I achieved an even higher level of trust. I not only trusted myself and my baby, I trusted that the Universe itself was conspiring on my behalf, for all to go perfectly for me. It was like upgrading the trust that I had been living for years, to a new space. I never knew that my trust for the process of birth could grow, but it did! I understood my power more and took full responsibility for creating Ivy's birth; I was also grateful for it, because I learned so much from the experience.

For my last pregnancy, I thought about what I wanted for my birth with Orion–not what I didn't want. This mindset and focus changed so much for me. I ate what tasted good, exercised in a way that felt right, and enjoyed doing things that brought me joy.

With my other pregnancies, I did what others told me to do because they were natural recommendations. I ate a certain amount of protein every day, I walked twice a day (even though I hated doing that), and I did Kegel exercises, relentlessly. I did the things that I'd read about, throughout my pregnancies, because the ideas were from a natural perspective, and because I thought it was what I was supposed to do. I threw my trust in others who had walked a more natural path than the mainstream.

However, much of what I did during my previous three pregnancies weren't things that I enjoyed. Once I experienced a new birth paradigm, and how important feeling good truly was, I was able to tap into an even more natural and authentic place, within myself.

It didn't look or sound like anything I had ever read or heard about pregnancy or birth before–even in the most trusting, empowering groups that I had been part of. This aspect of combining birth, with awareness that your thoughts create your reality, is *revolutionary*; and it is something that has changed my outlook on so many things–even things that I had previously learned and taught as a natural childbirth educator and Doula. I was thinking in new ways and blazing trails that had never been blazed in childbirth education!

At this time in my life, I am happy to share this with others. Since creating *Sexy Birth* five years ago, I have been able to see the amazing experiences of hundreds of couples, whom I have worked with. Empowering women to make choices that best fit *who they are,* has dramatically shifted my work and practice as a birth professional.

Sexy Birth is an approach and perspective that completely personalizes the birth experience for the individual woman. It enables her to tap into her authenticity, and this, in itself, is the epitome of self-creation and joy. The focus on my work today, is empowering women to take full responsibility for their births, by taking full responsibility for their thoughts.

The birth of my fourth child, my son, Orion, was nothing like the others. Sure, the others had been life-changing, empowering and beautiful; but none of them were built on the idea that I create my birth reality, from the inside out. This means, *my thoughts about birth become my reality and experience.*

This is a powerful way to *truly* take full responsibility for your pregnancy and birth. Creating my birth from a place of pure happiness was such a profound awakening for me, as a woman and as a birth advocate. It made me realize why my other three births went exactly as they did.

Orion was born into this world in pure joy and peace. I labored alone and birthed him into this world exactly the way that I wanted and envisioned, painlessly and easily. He was eleven pounds, just like his sister; but this time, the experience was pure, *sexy*, bliss.

I knew that I could create a painless, fun and easy birth, once I knew the secret of controlling my thoughts. I learned if I didn't do this, negativity and fear could easily creep in and begin to create an experience that I didn't want–just like with Ivy's birth. The default cultural settings would take over my mind, and my birth would be created from this space of unfocused fear, rather than the controlled mindset of my own focused intention.

Your thoughts and feelings about the birth literally create the birth itself. So what do you want for your birth? Really ask yourself this. Explore your desires and know there is no right or wrong answer. Begin to develop your own personal list of "wants" for your experience. Don't focus on the "don't wants" because the focus on those will bring them closer to you. Begin to shift all of your attention to your *desires* and bring your personal trust to a new level!

After giving birth to Orion, I knew that his birth was so profound, because I took the responsibility of birth into a new awareness.

Sexy Birth

2

SENSUAL HEALTH

Being pregnant is a unique and emotionally intense time for most women. Your hormones are fluctuating and so are your moods. You can feel extremely joyful one moment, and then crash with fear the next. It is a time of contemplation and growth. When you surround yourself with supportive, positive individuals, you are helping to create the experience you desire. When you have negative people around you, this affects the pregnancy and birth, profoundly.

If there are negative, fearful people in your life, pregnancy offers a time to rethink relationships. Do you want your baby to be born into this community of negativity, when you can actively choose a better one? Do you take the responsibility to focus on all that is working in your relationships, to help the positivity of your experience grow? Even if you do have people in your life that you feel you can't get away from, you can choose your thoughts about them. You can focus on your commonalities, and begin to be the type of person that you have always admired.

When you get together with others, you can choose to think about what you love or appreciate about them. Maybe your mother-in-law is a controlling, judgmental woman, but you love her cooking; or maybe you appreciate the ways in which she *does* support you. When you choose to consciously focus on what is working in your current relationships, even those that seem dysfunctional, you will be amazed how quickly the people in your life change. Or do they? When YOU change, your reality and perceptions about others change too. Personal growth shifts so much in your life.

Try focusing on what you love about others, not what you don't like, and see what it does for your life. You will be amazed at the results.

Throughout pregnancy, everyone around you will give advice on what to eat, what not to eat, what kind of activities to take part in and which ones are "dangerous". You hear everyone's opinions and suggestions, whether you like it or not. The truth about creating a healthy pregnancy is to do what feels good to you, and only you. No one else can tell you what that is. When you tune into your body's needs, more than likely, you will gravitate to a healthy, varied diet. You will just naturally want to move at times, and at other times, rest.

You begin a partnership with your child by listening and respecting his needs when he is in utero. You do this by responding to cravings and tuning into your body. If you want ice cream every day, eat it! If you crave a week-long binge on tomatoes, listen to that inner voice that is telling you what you need in that moment. When you begin turning to others for advice, your inner voice becomes unclear.

While pregnant, it is hard to trust your inner knowing and your baby, if every book, family member, friend and professional is telling you that they know better than you do. This is *your* body and *your* baby, and now is the time to tap into your instincts and inner knowing about what is best for you.

When you begin listening, your instinct grows stronger and louder. By the time your baby is born, you will be in such alignment with his needs that mothering will be easy and joyful for you–just as it was intended to be!

If you are eating foods that you don't enjoy because you think that you *should* be eating them, they aren't doing you any good *at all*. In fact, they are doing the opposite for your body and your baby.

Everything in the universe is made up of energy. You and your thoughts are made up of energy too. If you eat something you don't enjoy, that food is marinating in negative energy because of your feelings surrounding it. When you consume something that you don't like, you consume this negativity, which is never good for you.

I know this may sound really strange the first time you hear it, but it is scientifically proven: eating ice cream in pure bliss and gratitude is *better for you, physically,* than eating a carrot in guilt and obligation!

During my first three pregnancies, I gained between eighty and one hundred pounds with each pregnancy! I had borderline gestational diabetes as well, and I never ate anything that others would say was "bad" for me–no coffee, no ice cream or chocolate. I ate nothing that I wasn't "supposed" to and adhered to the high-protein diet, recommended by my midwives. As a childbirth educator, this was what I taught and promoted for years!

There were so many foods that I choked down every day, foods that I was told I should be eating. I was told to consume 80 to 100 grams of protein *every single day*. Years later, I learned that with my small frame, I needed *much less* than the average woman needed in order to sustain and nurture a healthy pregnancy. To put every woman on the same "pregnancy diet" is just wrong and dangerous. Why didn't I see or understand this before?!

During my *aware* pregnancy with Orion, I was able to tap into a part of myself that knew what I *really* wanted and needed. I was able to sit and feel the cravings that I had and actually act on them, instead of resist them.

I spread almond butter on apples and celery and ate a lot of fresh fruit. I enjoyed mostly living, raw foods; but also, when I craved it, I enjoyed quesadillas with gooey cheese–my favorite! I ate raw chocolate and enjoyed my morning cup of organic coffee, every day. I lived in a space of loving what I was eating, always, and through feeling good, I found my own balance. I trusted myself in a new way and as a result, Orion was grown with the optimal nutrition, health and happiness possible!

Everything that went into my body was with pure love and *positive energy*. As a result, I gained only a fraction of the weight that I did with my other pregnancies, and I had so much more joy and energy to live life to the fullest! This was, of course, helpful with three other young children who needed me to be at my best. I could connect with them with abundant, loving energy and enthusiasm!

A diet with as many living, whole foods as possible seemed to be what I was most drawn to. The enzymes in live, raw foods gave me so much energy and sense of well-being, every day! *Superfood* smoothies, fruits, veggies, nuts, sprouted whole grains, and raw cacao desserts were a big part of my diet during my last pregnancy. Instead of eating by a chart or "pregnancy diet," I ate with my heart–perfectly individualized pregnancy nutrition! I was healthier and happier than I had ever felt before!

These *high-vibe* foods give your body and baby all that you need for a healthy pregnancy. I never forbid myself anything and had no agenda, other than respecting my instinct to give my body and baby what they needed to grow healthy and strong.

I ate what tasted good, without referring to charts, professionals or books. My diet was balanced and varied. I never limited myself, counted protein or controlled my desires for things deemed "bad" for me. I respected my cravings and desires as an extension of myself; and this self-love for all of my choices brought me to a new level of understanding about diet during pregnancy.

The results were astounding. I gained much less weight, but still had a healthy eleven pound baby! I was healthier than I had ever been, because I trusted myself and acted on instinct. I was finally in alignment with my true self and it was delightful!

I want you to know that you will be at your healthiest during your pregnancy, if you honor what tastes good to you. Listen to your body, and as you eat whatever you choose, enjoy every minute of it!

Do not feel guilty when eating something you were told is bad for you. If you do, it becomes a self-fulfilling prophecy, because the food will be infused with guilt, fear and negativity. If you feel gratitude and joy when you eat, however, this is what you will be putting into your body. It will nourish you, sustain you and grow your baby with positive energy –filled with love, joy and bliss!

Sexy Birth

3

SEXERCISE!

Let your feelings be your guide! In regard to
exercise during pregnancy, this is the most
important piece of information that I share
with women: instead of looking at it as
"exercise," just look at it as "living an active
life."

There are some things that you can do to help
prepare your body for labor and birth.
Squatting is one thing that is helpful. Learning
to squat can help prepare your body for labor
and birth, by simply getting your body used to
this natural position. In our culture, however,

we don't do much squatting, so it is something we need to practice.

Squatting is an easy position to birth in. By squatting during pregnancy, you get your body used to that position in case you decide to use it during labor. It shortens the birth canal and significantly opens the pelvis. The pushing time is shorter and more comfortable when you squat.

If squatting feels uncomfortable for you, don't do it! You should *only* do what feels good to you. If you are an active person by nature, don't worry about starting a new exercise routine just because you are pregnant. Just carry on with your life, as you did before you were pregnant.

I know a lot of students who started yoga once they found out they were pregnant, because yoga was the "thing to do" among the circles they were part of. Most of them loved yoga, but some found it slow and boring. They found much greater satisfaction swimming, light weight training or dancing!

Some of my students disliked exercise altogether. In that case, I told them not to put too much pressure on themselves about it; because if they didn't enjoy whatever they were doing, it wouldn't do them any good, anyway. Instead, I asked them what brought them *joy* in life. One of them said "shopping." When I suggested shopping in the mall for exercise, she smiled. She found her blissful exercise, and she was able to have a healthy, joyful pregnancy because she felt good about the way she chose to be active!

Kegels are old school! The whole idea surrounding them is something you can let go of! They will actually make birth more *difficult.*

Doing Kegels all the time will get you a TIGHT, ineffective pelvic floor. Yes, this is mind-blowing to read, but it is well-documented and researched. Squatting is much more effective than doing Kegels. I have witnessed women who have done Kegels religiously during pregnancy (because they were recommended), have very difficult pushing stages because the muscles were too tight! You don't have to do them like you are lifting weights. It isn't natural for birth! Relaxed, loose, naturally developed muscles are much better for birth. The Kegel fad is behind us! Squatting is the natural exercise to lengthen and strengthen the pelvic floor muscles in a balanced, natural way.

So as you can see, maintaining a healthy pregnancy isn't as black and white as you have been led to believe. Just because you think something is natural and healthy, doesn't mean it is for *you*, as an individual. The clients that I worked with, who listened to their instincts and trusted their desires (what felt good and right to them in any given moment), were the most healthy and happy pregnancies. These resulted in amazingly joyful births. The most natural, healthy and joyful births are the result of the mother being her most authentic self. This is the epitome of a natural, *Sexy Birth.*

Robin Elise Weiss, LCCE shares:

"Sex during pregnancy is healthy and natural. It isn't discussed very much because of the cultural tendency of not associating expectant mothers with sexuality. When we see pregnancy as the pinnacle of sexuality that it is, you can understand how sex during pregnancy can be very pleasurable and important.

There are many reasons why sex during pregnancy, can be even more enjoyable than it was before you were pregnant. There is an increase in vaginal lubrication and engorgement of the genital area. This helps some women become orgasmic for the first time or multi-orgasmic for the first time! The lack of birth control–or if you have been trying for a while–a return to sex as pleasure (as opposed to being only for procreation), and other factors, can allow for a new and relaxed approach to your sexuality as a couple.

Change what you view as a normal, healthy pregnancy–both in your body and your beliefs. While some women may feel large and uncomfortable, men generally find the pregnant body very erotic and desirable.

Make sure that you discuss the feelings that you have about sex and sexuality. These discussions can lead to a more fulfilling sex life. If either of you do not feel like having sex, this can be particularly important. Explain to your partner what is going on and what they can do to help you be sexual. Here are some examples: more cuddling, relaxing baths, romantic dinners, massages and mutual masturbation. Whatever you and your partner agree upon is exactly what you need.

The hormonal fluctuations and trimesters of pregnancy also play a part in your reactions to making love. Many women are too fatigued and nauseated to be very interested during the first trimester–while the second trimester can bring a new sense of delight as your belly grows. The third trimester can be a fun time to get really creative with positions during sex. It is a good idea to keep a supply of water-based lubricant". (The full article by Robin Elise Weiss called, "Sex During Pregnancy What You Need to Know" can be found on About.com)

Semen is also very beneficial during pregnancy. During late pregnancy, the semen can help soften the cervix and get it ripe for birth. It will not put you into labor unless your body is truly ready.

"Semen is good stuff. It gives a shot of zinc, calcium, potassium, fructose, proteins -- a veritable cornucopia of vitality! Some studies show that semen acts like an antidepressant for many women because of its amazing qualities. It can also help with morning sickness, boost cardio health and lower blood pressure.

Another recent study found that women who gave their men oral sex, and swallowed, had a lower risk of preeclampsia, the dangerously high blood pressure that sometimes accompanies pregnancy. Evidence also shows that the vagina absorbs a number of components of semen, which can be detected in the bloodstream within a few hours of its consumption.

An orgasm is a powerful pain-killer! Oxytocin –a natural chemical in the body that surges before and during climax– gets some of the credit, along with endorphins and a couple of other compounds.

According to a study by famous sexologist and author Beverly Whipple, when women masturbated to orgasm, "the pain tolerance threshold and pain detection threshold increased significantly by 74.6 percent and 106.7 percent respectively." This is why masturbating during pregnancy, and especially during labor, will be so beneficial! (If your water has broken already, be sure to only give yourself clitoral stimulation during labor.)

Enjoying an orgasm during pregnancy does much to calm you, whether alone or with a partner. It helps with sleep for many women who are experiencing restlessness, due to physical and emotional changes". Brian Alexander (NBC 2006 from the article, "Not just good, but good for you").

It is normal and healthy to be the beautiful, sexual being that you truly are, during this special time in your life. Do what makes you comfortable and enjoy every minute of it! This can be a time of great connection and exploration, for both you and your partner!

4

HURTS SO GOOD!

Pain. When a woman is pregnant, just the word can bring up some intense emotions. There is so much fear surrounding birth and pain. We have been led to believe that pain is essential to bringing forth life. The pain of childbirth, however, isn't *really* pain at all. If a woman has never given birth the sensations can be overwhelming and unpleasant, especially if she isn't aware of what to do with her body and mind during labor.

However, pain *isn't* the word I would use to describe the sensations of a normal birth. Incredible, raw, powerful, and intense, best describes what birth is like when a woman is in a state of allowing.

When you resist these sensations, it *can* hurt. All of the muscles in your body are connected. Your uterus is a huge bag of muscles, and even tensing your hands can start a tug-of-war with your body's process of birthing. When you resist, pain persists! Being conscious of the fact that tension causes your muscles to contract, and resist contractions, can help you understand how truly important *allowing* is during labor.

Negative emotion causes pain during labor and birth. It is *so* important to stay as positive and confident as you can. It is in a state of *allowing and welcoming*, that a woman can have a positive birth experience, and bring a baby into this world in pure joy.

Birth becomes so much easier when you can be in a confident, happy and even *sexy* place, mentally, during your labor. Pain takes a back seat, and by allowing and welcoming the intense energy of contractions, it can all be simple and even pleasurable!

This may be like nothing you have ever heard before regarding birth, but it is *real* and it is *true*. The average woman can experience birth as sensual, easy, joyful and fun. I've witnessed it myself, over and over again, while working with women in my classes and attending their births. Your only job is to feel good!

What you have been led to believe about birth are all myths and lies that have been perpetuated. However, I have seen an amazing shift in our culture–even Pampers has a commercial showing a woman having a home water birth! Times are changing, and we are evolving to understand how birth is meant to be for families. I love the progress and growth, taking place in our world right now, and I am so honored to be part of it all.

So how does a woman have one of these empowering, intense, but beautiful

experiences? She s*tops thinking about pain.*
Whenever you get scared about birth, instead
of trying to *not* think about your fear, do
something that brings you joy! Listen to your
favorite music or read a powerful, inspiring
poem. Eat something you love or go out for a
walk. You need to actively *do* something to
shift your inner thoughts.

Sometimes you can just sit and allow yourself
to feel the depths of that fear, without needing
to judge it in any way. You can step out of
yourself for a moment, and realize that you are
not your fear. Take a look at it and say, "Isn't
this interesting that I am feeling so fearful right
now. Hmmm… I wonder why?" If you can't
shift your feelings, don't resist them. Feel them
deeply and allow them to move through you.

You can really feel it and own it, and once you
do this, you can move on–instead of feeling
like it is somehow wrong to be feeling fearful.
Don't make it such heavy burden though. Just
be light with it all and look at it, and just
observe your emotions without judgment.

"Huh… fear. I wonder what triggered that?" Don't resist this part of who you are, either. Allow it all during this time in your life. It is a very healthy, natural way to deal with what you are experiencing.

There are things that women do to create *unnecessary* pain during their labor. This is important to discuss, because when you know what *not* to do, it can allow you to shift to a place of confidence in your ability to birth your baby. This confidence allows space for you to feel how your body works during labor and birth.

It is so important to be rested before your labor, as it requires your *complete* focus. If you do go into labor in the middle of the night, the best thing you can do is go back to sleep! I know this can be hard because you are so excited, but you don't know if your labor is going to be hours or days (either of which is normal); and being tired is *not* conducive to an easy, joyful birth experience.

Labor and birth are like an athletic event. What would happen if pro-athletes didn't sleep before their big Olympic event? You guessed it… they wouldn't do very well and would not be at their peak, mentally or physically. You know how cranky you are when you are tired. Can you imagine what birthing like that would be like? So, at the very least, rest if you can, and ideally, sleep until the labor needs more of your attention. You'll know when that is. Nature will tell you.

Eating during labor is also very important, especially if early labor is long. Looking back at the athletes, can you imagine how their performances would be if they didn't eat, the whole day before they competed? Again, they wouldn't perform very well. They would be run down and tired and *not* in a very joyful place. I know I am a total misery to be around if I am hungry! You aren't very balanced emotionally when your body is depleted, so eating whatever tastes good to you is exactly what you should be doing.

There was a time in my professional education, when I heard that eating carbohydrates were preferable for a laboring woman; but depending on your body type and what you are craving, it may *not* be ideal. This is why I say that simply eating what tastes good to you is the best choice for your experience.

I did lean toward whole, fresh foods during my labors; but I distinctly remember having a few yummy bites of chocolate, in between contractions, with my last birth. It really raised my energetic vibration and it tasted SO good, which made me really happy; and being in that state during labor is the best space you can be in.

Drinking water and juice during labor is something you will just want to do, naturally. Water is the basis of human functioning and without it, your uterus doesn't contract as efficiently, and you are not at your peak physical state. Some people love Gatorade during labor. I enjoyed 100% fruit juice and water–A LOT of water. You sweat so much during pushing, that you lose a ton of hydration. When I am with them during their births, I always make it a point to offer my clients water between every contraction.

When you are drinking so much water during labor, you should be going to the bathroom often. A full bladder causes so much unnecessary pain during labor! Most of the time women think that it is the pain of the labor itself that is causing so much discomfort. Because so much is going on physically, it is hard to distinguish between certain sensations. When you have a contraction with a full bladder, it hurts!

I once arrived at a birth, only to see a mother in bed, hollering in pain. She was asking me why it felt like it did, because she felt she was doing everything "right." I reminded her to go empty her bladder, and once she did, she came out of the bathroom with a huge grin on her face. She said, "I'm so glad you were here to remind me about that! I feel so much better!" I wonder how many women labor in pain, thinking the pain is caused by labor itself; when in actuality, it is simply a need to go to the bathroom!

If you happen to be laboring in a birthing tub or shower and you have to pee, just go in the tub. Seriously! Urine is sterile and there is no harm to you or the baby from doing that. It is so diluted and no one will ever know, unless you announce it. It is safe, common and encouraged.

Walking is another wonderful way to naturally focus on pleasure. Lying in bed on your back is the worst possible position to birth in. The reason we see it so often in the media, is because over 90% of women choose medication during their labors. When you do this, the only position you are allowed to be in, is usually in bed, on your back.

Historically, it is easier for a doctor to deliver that way, and being a business, hospitals like to do things in the best interests of their employees. So the supine position is culturally, the norm. It is also the most painful, unnatural position to be in when pushing a baby out.

What is so interesting is that the pain many women experience in labor, is caused simply by how birth is managed. A woman feels pain from being told to lie on her back, and then the pain meds are given– which then keep a woman on her back. It seems really ridiculous, but since such a majority of women choose to go this route, the myth of pain during childbirth is perpetuated, over and over again. I want you to know that what you have been conditioned to believe about birth, is simply not true and doesn't resemble what normal birth looks like. Release any ideas you may have had in the past, and open your mind to learning about another reality: the reality of those bringing their babies into this world with peace, joy and love.

When you are lying on your back and have a contraction, your uterus moves forward and your baby's head hits the pelvic bones over and over again, causing a great deal of pain for the mother and baby. After hours of these negative sensations, the baby may move up and over the bones to be born, but it isn't without incident. Often times the babies heart rate will drop, especially if medication is given. Panic sets in when this happens, and a Cesarean birth is ordered.

The incredible part of the whole ordeal is that the mother ends up thanking the well-intentioned professionals for saving her baby, when they were the ones that actually caused the problems by the way they managed the birth!

There are certain things you can do every day, to help prepare for the experience of labor and birth. You can help increase your stamina and flexibility, so birth goes smoothly and easily.

Squatting is a common position in most cultures around the world. We aren't necessarily used to squatting, but it is a position that is fabulous to birth in! As I mentioned, it shortens the birth canal and opens your pelvis so the baby can slip through, easily and smoothly.

If you are someone who doesn't squat, now would be a great time to start! Instead of bending over to pick things up, squat down to get your body and muscles ready for birth. Watch television or read in the squatting position, and increase your time every day.

You may end up pushing in this position for hours, which is normal for first time mothers. If your body isn't prepared for that possibility, it won't be an option for you. So prepare your body now to open up your options! You will be glad you did!

Whatever exercise appeals to you during pregnancy, is what you should be doing–not what a doctor, midwife or someone else suggests–only what YOU want to do. Some women love walking, swimming, hiking or shopping! It is all up to you. The important thing is to try to remain active, because building and maintaining your stamina will keep your spirits and energy high. This is exactly what you want to maintain for your present happiness, as well as the energy you'll need during labor.

Go for regular massages! It is a pleasurable way to keep your circulation flowing perfectly and for you to get used to receiving pleasure. You deserve it and you are worthy; so if you enjoy massages, make it an important, regular appointment during pregnancy. A massage appointment is just as important as a prenatal appointment! Taking good care of yourself, in this way, is something you should get used to for both your physical and emotional health.

Your child will learn how to *be* in this world from how you yourself are living. When you show them you are worthy of good self-care and nurturing, they learn to care and nurture themselves too. Our children do not learn from how we tell them to be. They learn from our modeling. Be good to yourself and your kids will be good to themselves, too. If you can't do it for yourself, do it for your child.

When it comes to nutrition and exercise during pregnancy, the important thing to remember is not to take it all too seriously. Eat well and joyfully. Move with love and purpose. Think good quality thoughts about birth. Enjoy the process and savor every moment. You will look back at this time as pivotal in learning how to trust and allow. This time is sacred, and it should be fun and pleasurable.

 Don't get caught up in being too serious or melancholy with it all. This part of your life– well, *every* part of your life–is supposed to be amazing and playful! Smile and know that all is well, as much as you can. Your baby will only benefit from being grown with such joyful energy surrounding him.

Labor doesn't have to be painful. There are many things you can do to prevent the unnecessary pain– that most in our culture think is all part of the process. If I didn't share anything else with you but this one chapter, your birth would already be so much more positive and more pleasurable than most women and most birth professionals ever learn it can be! From reading what you've read so far, you now know more about natural birth than most nurses and doctors ever learn in their entire careers! I hope that knowing this brings you to a new level of confidence.

We tend to accept our beliefs as fact. "Childbirth is painful," is one belief that many of us have accepted: but I am writing to share that this isn't *fact*. It is not my truth, nor does it have to be yours. I have experienced a painless childbirth and–it is not only possible–it is what most women in tribal cultures experience. When you can open your mind and begin researching for yourself that painless birth is possible and desirable, you have a much better chance at creating that experience for yourself. When you hold on to the belief that pain is inevitable during birth, you will create that for yourself as well.

A belief is only a thought that you have been thinking, over and over again. You can adopt new beliefs, simply by thinking new thoughts! "Birth does not have to be painful," is one of the beliefs you can take on. It won't be a possibility for you, unless you believe it to be true!

Immersing yourself in the growing community of women, who are having amazing, joyful births, is the first step in reprogramming your mind to form different beliefs. You need to un-brainwash yourself to think of birth in a certain way! This takes time and effort, but it will be easy and fun, once you step into this whole new way of looking at birth. Do a search online for painless birth, and see what you learn and what you create for yourself. The time to shift your beliefs is now, and in doing so, your entire reality and experience will reflect your new perspective.

Positive beliefs and attitudes contribute to a positive and joyful birth experience. If you believe your body is designed to birth easily and effectively, it will!

5

PASSIONATE CONSUMERISM

This is something I love to share with the couples that I work with: The people you decide to hire to help during your pregnancy, labor and birth, are working FOR you. Whom you decide to surround yourself with has a profound effect on your entire experience. You never have to listen to any information or advice over listening to your own instinct.

The doctors, nurses, midwives, doulas and childbirth educators are all people you are paying to serve you. Their role shouldn't be to scare you into doing what *they* think you should be doing. It is great to weigh options and choices, but ultimately, you are the one who has the last say in everything. You need to self-design your birth.

Not everyone wants to take this responsibility during this sacred time in their lives. Sometimes women like to hire people to make all of the decisions for them. Often, as a result, they end up having very negative experiences because they never stepped up and researched what options best suited them and their own, unique beliefs surrounding pregnancy and birth. This mindset of taking no responsibility, often leads couples to blame and feel victimized–which is a cultural default mindset that most of us were raised in. It feels comfortable to let everyone else make all of the decisions for us; but it is usually not fulfilling or satisfying to allow your experience to be managed by someone else, who puts their own agendas and needs first. You may be an important client or patient, but never assume your needs and desires will be put before theirs. It just doesn't work that way.

Taking full responsibility for your birth is your first step in being a powerful creator in your life. Deciding what you want and then taking the necessary steps to get it, takes more effort than simply being pushed through the machine of what everyone else does. When you take the responsibility to self-design your birth, your experience will not be like the experience of the majority of women in our culture. It is a powerful feeling to know you can create the birth you want, by carefully hand-selecting who will be educating you, supporting you and uplifting you.

Do you want to birth in a hospital, home, or birth center? Do you want a doctor, midwife, or doula? Do you want to have an unassisted birth, where only you and your partner bring forth your baby, on the same continuum of sensuality in which your creation began? *There are no wrong choices*. There is only what YOU want. You will hear a barrage of opinions and beliefs surrounding birth, along the way. Your best chance for a positive, healthy and joyful experience will be to create the experience that you feel is best for *you*, as an individual.

If you choose a hospital birth, your best chance to have a normal, natural experience is to hire a doula. A doula will ensure that your birth wishes are respected and she serves to support you in the way you want to be supported. If you don't have a doula in the hospital, you will have labor support, whether you want it or not, but it will be from the nurse that happens to be on duty. This is like going on a blind date. Most nurses *aren't* familiar with normal, natural birth, and their suggestions and style of support often undermine your desires. They were trained in the medical management of birth, not the allowing that is necessary for a natural birth.

It can be really tough if you do not have someone there who knows you and your personal birth philosophy. If money is an issue, most midwifery students will serve as a doula for free, to get some births under their belt– which is a requirement of their training. In addition, some doulas will barter for services. No matter how fabulous your partner or friends are, they are never a replacement for a doula, in a hospital setting. Be a good consumer, in this regard, and do the leg-work necessary to surround yourself with people who are trusting, confident and who share the same philosophy that you do, about birth.

Call several doulas and chat with them on the phone. Get a feel for who is a good match for you. Some you will click with and others you will not. *Do not just go by a friend's recommendation.* Really take the time to meet with different doulas to find someone you are really comfortable with. Choose a doula that feels like a friend and who is upbeat and joyful in their demeanor.

Some doulas are really serious and carry a heavy, fearful energy. They may have a very anti-hospital and intervention stance. This negative energy will be carried to your birthing experience and it may conflict with your energy, and that of the hospital staff.

Sometimes this type of doula carries with her a lot of fear of the hospital institution. If this is the case, your birth team may view her as antagonistic, and a power struggle may ensue. You do not need any negative energy at your birth! Make sure your doula is loving, kind and warm in her energy. Not all doulas are the same, so do your research and hire the best match for who you are, and what you hope to create for yourself and your baby.

Many of my students start off assuming they will have a hospital birth, only to change their mind half-way through the class series. Once they truly understand the safety of homebirth and they see that more and more women are choosing homebirth, they begin to rethink their beliefs surrounding it.

At my first prenatal appointment when I found out I was pregnant with my second child, my hospital-based midwife suggested that I have a homebirth, since my first birth went so beautifully. She told me that she'd had all of her babies at home. I was stunned at the suggestion. I never knew anyone who had their babies at home! A new world that I'd never considered was opened to me, and it changed my life forever.

I called a team of homebirth midwives to make an appointment as soon as I got home. I felt so nervous meeting them, because I didn't think that I would fit in with the alternative vibe of the homebirth world. Much to my surprise, they were some of the kindest and coolest women that I have ever met! Joe had so many questions about emergency situations. One of them was, "What if Dayna needs a Cesarean?" They calmly explained the rare instances in which it would be necessary, and what they would do to handle it. Instantly, we felt relaxed and educated about each and every scenario, in case a variation of normal birth occurred.

The midwives shared that they bring all of the equipment that hospitals use for emergencies, with them to homebirths, and they are highly trained in normal birth as well as variations. On the ride home, Joe and I grew so excited! I never pictured myself as a homebirther! It was a new identity, and one that I was so proud to embrace.

During the time that I was planning my first homebirth, I was also studying to be a childbirth educator and doula, myself. I was learning about the safety of homebirth for my training and my personal experience, simultaneously. I was living my passion on every level and was completely in alignment with my true self.

My natural birth with my second child was very profound. My daughter, Dakota, came into this world in a way that I wanted everyone to experience, but something was lacking. I allowed loving spectators–my mother-in-law and sister-in-law–to just sit and watch me birth. It affected the experience in a way that I wasn't prepared for.

I later learned that a woman, simply being observed during labor, is much like a woman being observed during sex. Can you imagine your mother-in-law being there to witness the conception of your child? The same feeling is present during labor and birth, when people are there purely to watch the baby come into this world.

Having them there felt so peculiar and made me really hold back. I was not able to turn inward–where I needed to turn–to allow for a joyful birth. Consequently, I experienced more pain than I would have if I was alone, or just with those taking an active role in the process. I was embarrassed, withdrawn and self-conscious. Those emotions should never be present during the birth of your child.

As a fear-driven childbirth educator and doula, I was very well-intentioned. I knew that fear was an incredible motivator and I *did* have an agenda. I believed that a natural birth was best for every woman and every child. My ego took the front seat and I wanted my students and clients to achieve the birth that *I* thought they should have. I felt successful and important if I achieved that goal while assisting them.

To motivate them to birth in a way that I thought was best, I showed my students videos of how scary a Cesarean could be. I showed babies separated from their mothers, and women being strapped down in birthing beds. I focused on that kind of education for many years. It was how I was trained to teach as a childbirth educator!

Then I had my third birthing experience, and began to rethink everything that I thought about childbirth education and support. I experienced something that would change me on every level as I walked my own path as a woman, advocate, educator and mother.

When my third child, Ivy, was born posterior, it was very traumatic for me. There was no joy in the experience at all, except when it was finally over. I began to wonder if my goal for a natural birth should outweigh the goal of a *Joyful Birth*. My past beliefs began to unravel, and I allowed myself to stand in a place of deep questioning of my beliefs, in what the ultimate goal of birth should be.

Is a natural childbirth more important than a joyful childbirth? If a variation comes up, is medication and intervention one way in which more joy and pleasure can enter the experience?

I was so happy that I *did* birth Ivy at home; but in my situation–the rare experience of an over ten pound posterior delivery–could I have experienced more joy and less trauma, by having Ivy in the hospital? Or would that decision have left me with even more emotional and physical scars, given the risks associated with surgery? I will never know. All I can do is be grateful for the experience as it offered me so much insight and personal growth.

I never regret what I went through with Ivy's birth because it enabled me to shift in my beliefs, and become a better educator and doula. Little did I know how much this shift would propel me in a new direction, toward an entirely different birth paradigm and educational perspective–one that I could share with millions of women all over the world!

I think for the majority of women, a homebirth, and even an unassisted birth is not only possible, it is the *best chance* for the most joyful and healthy experience for both mother and baby. I also feel that a joyful and healthy experience in the hospital can be possible, but not if the woman is making the choice to birth there out of fear. If fear is part of the equation, I think she should at least meet with some homebirth midwives and discuss the option.

I also think a woman can be scared into birthing at home, when childbirth education and support is focused on an agenda–rather than the woman's individual needs and desires.

When a woman is designing her own birth, she should ask herself what feels best to her when looking at the options. No one should ever judge her choice or try to sway her because of his or her own fears. Where she births is the choice of the individual woman, and her feelings are what will create the experience and outcome.

If the partner is feeling nervous about homebirth but the expectant Mom is desiring one, it is the *responsibility of the partner* to do their research, to aid in making a truly informed decision, as a couple. A partner should never try to control the expectant mother and become the authority. It is important to research the options together, in complete partnership, so both of you feel good about wherever you choose to have your baby.

There is so much misinformation out there about hospitals, birth centers *and* homebirths. To truly be a good consumer, you need to take the time to personalize your own unique experience. Visit the hospital, birth centers and meet with homebirth midwives. Most people spend much more time planning their wedding than they ever do planning their birth. Take as much care in doing the planning and designing of the birth of your child. It is, after all, the most sacred of human experiences!

If anyone attending the birth is fearful about it, bringing the fearful or negative energy to the birth itself is not wise. It will definitely affect the woman's experience if her partner is the one full of fear. Couples are usually very closely connected during this time, so his state of being has the potential to affect the quality of the birth experience, in a very deep way.

The energy surrounding the birthing woman is easily felt by her during labor. She picks it up like a lightning rod, and she is very vulnerable and sensitive to any shift in energy. As a doula, it is my job to hold the space for the laboring woman; I ensure that everyone takes full responsibility for the energy that they bring into her birthing space.

This is something that not many expectant couples or even birth professionals consider, when they think about birth. The energy, or the non-physical aspect of the experience, is just as important as the physical. As a doula, it isn't just about massage and encouraging words. It is about minding your energy and feelings, and taking the responsibility to maintain the positive and joyful energy, conducive to birthing in peace and love. It is so much more than what we learn in our childbirth education training.

Supporting your partner on their own path as they learn about birth is just as important as your learning about it, yourself. Helping them see how safe and joyful birth can be, can be a real source of connection for you both. Your partner's role during the experience is not usually respected in the birthing community, to the level that I believe it should be.

He is being born a father during this time, and the three of you are being born a family. Your partner may not be physically experiencing the same thing you are, but emotionally, he is going through his own evolution. He should also be honored and respected during your labor. It is something he will always remember; how he was treated during the experience will always stay with him.

I have witnessed a fearful and unsupportive partner relax in the waiting room, while his partner labored with a doula present, supporting her through hard labor. He had a lot of anxiety and because of this he couldn't come to a place of trust with labor and birth. For her to have the safest and healthiest birth possible, he opted to stay out of the birthing space, until she was pushing. He joined his wife in the birthing room just as their baby's head was crowning. He was able to witness and be part of the joyful, positive energy of the actual birth of his child, without affecting the labor negatively. This is something they worked out together, after considering their unique experience. They took the responsibility to self-design the best birth for *them*.

I am not suggesting this for all couples with this issue, but I was impressed with their ability to find a scenario that everyone was comfortable with, so that supportive energy was surrounding the woman during the labor. It was a win-win decision.

When peace and joy are priority, it leads to a positive outcome. There is always a way to get exactly what you want in your own unique birth, when considering all of your options. Sometimes thinking "outside the box" is necessary to create the birth you want.

Sexy Birth

6

YOUR SEXY LABOR

Most people think of labor as being one big chunk of time. Meaning, they have heard that labor begins and is broken up into stages, ever so neatly and linearly. The reality is that labor is usually something that happens over the course of several days, or even weeks.

For many women, labor begins and they have contractions for a couple of hours–and they are certain that it *is time!* They phone friends and family, who are all excitedly awaiting the arrival of their beautiful little being.

After a few hours, however, contractions seem to slow down. They go from being regular and gaining in strength, to dwindling away, even when the woman tries the things she has learned that might speed them up. Eventually the labor stops altogether, and the woman is left feeling frustrated and disappointed, like something must be wrong with her body.

The truth is, that experiencing labor like I described is very common and exactly what is supposed to happen! It is often just your body trying out contractions to see if you and the baby are ready for birth. It is *not* what is falsely labeled, "false labor." There is nothing *false* about it. In fact, that label is negative and leads women down a path of distrust of their bodies and of the processes of labor and birth. This starting and stopping is a completely common aspect of a normal labor.

It is such a shame that in a hospital setting, many caregivers will look at this as the woman's body being somehow broken or flawed. Drugs are given to "get things going more regularly," when it is only patience that is needed–not rushing the process through medical intervention.

When labor does stop after some time, it usually means that your body was not ready yet, or that the baby was not ready to be born yet. Maybe the baby's lungs weren't fully developed, or your muscles weren't quite ready. It isn't something you will ever know for sure, but it is important to just trust that it isn't quite time yet. What your body is doing is perfect and desirable, and a sign that the process of labor and birth are in true alignment.

When a caregiver messes with this delicate process to "get things going," it is not in the best interest of you or the baby, because nature *always* knows best. Your baby has grown perfectly inside you for the last nine or more months. To assume all of a sudden, that your body is "broken" will only cause problems that can rarely be fixed. For instance, if the baby needed a few more days for its lungs to mature, artificially speeding things up will put that baby at risk from intervention, once it is forced to be born.

Trusting the process and knowing in your heart that there is no such thing as *false labor,* is a step in the direction of partnership with your child and your body. With three of my four labors, this scenario played out just as I described. Homebirth midwives know how common this is, and mine didn't mind at all returning home after six hours of my laboring.

After hours with my contractions six minutes apart, my labor just stopped. I really appreciated the supportive, casual attitude of the midwives. They knew what true, natural labor is like. In a hospital setting, it would have been viewed as a problem, where intervention would have been insisted upon; because once you are there, you are on their clock to deliver under a certain amount of time.

Homebirth enabled me to allow my body and baby to work together, in love and trust of the normal process of birth. About four days later,

I went into labor again. I wasn't sure if it would stop or continue, so I just went about life until the labor switched gears into something more intense, and I knew it wasn't going to stop. At that point I called the midwives and they happily returned to attend my third birth. It was perfect that they encouraged me to just trust the process.

Laboring in joy is truly possible, but only if you understand a few things. Do not follow someone else's blueprint of how to birth! When I was planning my first homebirth, I read all of the books, did the exercises, and connected with other homebirthing Moms and birth professionals. I easily slipped into the homebirthing Mama identity. Hell, I even bought Birkenstocks!

I learned all of the ways in which I should be able to attain the ideal birth. It seemed that lavender candles (after all, lavender is the most relaxing scent) and listening to soft, relaxing music, like *Enya,* would be helpful. I was told that massage from my partner and gentle words of encouragement, whispered into my ear, would be what I needed. All of these scripted, common choices were what I thought would guarantee me my dream of a peaceful, natural home birth.

Much to my surprise, none of this really worked for me, personally, when birthing Dakota (my second child). The smell of lavender made me feel nauseated and the sound of *Enya* was so annoying to me as background music, that I was left feeling emotionally uncomfortable. Consequently, this led to physical discomfort. I wasn't able to communicate my needs in the throes of hard labor. I didn't want anyone to touch me, and by having so many people attend my birth, I somehow gave over my inner strength and power to them. My birth was amazing and powerfully transforming, but something was missing.

In the last decade of attending births, I have noticed an interesting phenomenon. The more people a woman has at her birth, the more power she gives over to them to support her, rather than her *herself* doing it. Subconsciously, because of their presence, she wants them to feel useful and fulfill *their* need and desire for being there. She trades her inner ability to birth perfectly, to make others happy and feel useful. Her strength is transformed into helplessness, as she reaches out to others, so their role and intention for being present is met.

I grew and evolved greatly from my second birth experience, because it offered so many insights. When I was pregnant the *third* time, I tried Native American chanting, instead of *Enya*, and I used a birthing tub. I found scented candles that I enjoyed, rather than using the kind I was told were relaxing. I changed my choices, and my new ideas were an upgrade from my prior birth experience, but I stayed within the old birthing paradigm–with a natural birth being the main goal and focus.

The entire experience of Ivy's birth turned out to be a swirl of confusion and desperation, just to birth her. Again, there were too many people there, touching me and trying to comfort me through the experience. I know they all had the most loving intentions, but all I really needed was to be alone to tap into my own needs, at that time.

After a very long, painful and intense experience, I *did* birth Ivy at home, so I was content with the outcome. However, the joy was greatly missing and this was something I never focused at all on when planning her birth. I never looked at birth through the lens of this new paradigm, where feeling good and being happy throughout labor and birth is the focus. I never gave myself the mental space to see that pleasure could be possible. I never created any of that for myself by just focusing on "natural" birth. Joyful, happy birth wasn't part of my reality, or my education and support of others. It was deeply focused and powerful intent on birthing *naturally*, but it ended there.

No matter where you choose to birth, the focus on feeling good, emotionally and physically, *needs* to be the priority, along with health and wellness. There needs to be *self-love, sensuality and trust* on the forefront of the creation and the goal of a joyful birth experience–no matter how the details work out, during the birth itself.

Planning the location, choosing care providers, and educating yourself and your partner about the logistics are all very important. Once these are all lined up though, you can let go and focus on the joy of being present and trusting the process. Feel yourself having a joyful, positive birth experience, and just take the full responsibility to simply feel good! *This* will line you up with a natural birth better than anything else you could possibly do.

So you see if you want a natural birth, you never have to follow someone else's idea of how to accomplish it. You do not need the intense education about the physical details of what your body will be doing during birth.

You don't need to know how electricity works to reap the benefits; and you don't need to know every detail about how everything will happen, physically, to be able to enjoy and welcome the experience. If anything, educating a couple by cramming them full of the information about the physical details of birth, takes away from the more important non-physical aspects, which are necessary to birth with *presence*.

In my own practice as a birth worker, I have learned that the focus should always be on how to help the mother *feel good and stay positive*, and the details will unfold in the most beautiful, organic way. Teaching about dilation, stages of labor and breathing exercises are old school and outdated. Focusing on feeling good and taking responsibility for the energy brought into the birthing space, is the leading-edge in childbirth education.

7

ROCK YOUR BIRTH!

Being authentically YOU is *sexy.* Birthing in your own way is something that is scary for most people, because they want a blueprint of how to do things. Natural birth isn't about making the same choices that the naturally-minded Moms, who've walked before you, have made. *Natural* is being true to yourself and what feels good to you, as an individual.

Creating my last birth experience with my son, Orion, by getting into true alignment with who I was as a woman, was essential in having the joyful and painless birth experience that I had.

I am glad that I have personally experienced and witnessed so many different births, to be able to bring this awareness to others. I am so happy to share what is possible when one takes responsibility for her own thoughts.

Many women never see birth as a continuum of sexuality. To have a joyful, painless birth, where you surrender completely, you really have to honor that it *is* a lot like having sex. Being alone or alone with your partner, is the best chance you have at experiencing a sensual, joyful, painless birth. Yes, your birth can be positive with an audience; but in order to reach higher levels of consciousness during birth, and to be able to tap into that part of yourself that is necessary to allow the vibration of sexuality to easily flow, birth shouldn't be a spectator event.

I like to share this analogy with the fathers that I work with: How well would you "perform" during lovemaking, with your mother in the room witnessing it? How about if you had doctors strapping monitors on you, asking you repeatedly if you were getting close to climaxing? What would the experience be like? I thought so... totally *un*sexy! It is the same for laboring women who are observed, frequently checked for dilation and monitored. It is just plain *harder* to give birth, in the same way as it would be to engage in intercourse, under the same conditions. It changes the entire experience–from joyful and positive, to embarrassing, painful and fearful.

If you are deeply set that your mother, friends or family witness the birth, I highly encourage you to have them wait in another room until the baby is actually crowning. Then you can have your partner or birth attendant go and get them to witness the actual *birth itself*. Having them present during hard labor and transition, makes the experience more uncomfortable and awkward for the laboring woman, especially if you are planning to ride the continuum of intimacy and connection with your partner, during the process.

Early labor is an incredible opportunity for couples to connect with one another, in a way that they will remember forever. It is a time to honor the true continuum of sexuality and sensuality that actually conceived your child to begin with! I didn't fully understand this continuum with my first three birth experiences. It wasn't until I began reading all that I could get my hands on about unassisted birth that I reached a new awareness of what birth could be.

I learned that women, who birthed alone or with their partners, could experience birth as pleasurable and sensual. It made perfect sense! As the famous midwife Ina May Gaskin says, *"The energy that gets the baby in, gets the baby out."* I had heard that so many times, but I never fully understood it to the core, until I myself experienced what birth could be like from this perspective.

I never experienced birth as a continuum of love or sexuality before my birth with Orion. Our culture views birth and sexuality as separate. When one thinks of birth, they generally think of it being medical, mechanical, painful and dangerous. I love to share that this doesn't have to be *your* reality! You can choose to have something very different than most woman experience; and in doing so, you will be getting in alignment with your child's birth to be as beautiful as their conception.

For my final birth, my plan was to have an unassisted, but *attended* birth. This means that I would be laboring and birthing alone, but that the midwives would be downstairs, in case I needed them. Due to the fact that I have large babies and I lose a significant amount of blood after giving birth, I tend to get faint. This is normal for some women. Joe's desire for assistance at the birth was an aspect of our self-designed experience.

We compromised by choosing to have back-up midwives here when I was giving birth, but that I would be upstairs laboring alone. My mother was also here, visiting from England, and she had never witnessed the birth of any of her grandchildren. I requested that she also wait until I called her to catch the baby.

My mother was so honored to be part of our own unique, perfectly orchestrated experience. I knew she was nervous and she knew that I wanted to be alone during hard labor and transition. She was more than respectful in my wishes and I am proud to say that she came in the room just in time to catch Orion as I pushed him into her hands. She was quite baffled when she saw him still in the amniotic sac and asked for my midwife to come up and help her remove the caul from his face. She had never witnessed a birth, and we laugh about how confused she was seeing him for the first time in a way that very few people have ever seen a baby be delivered–"en-caul"! It was absolutely incredible!

When labor began, everyone was in our living room, relaxing. Dakota and Ivy were asleep, but my oldest, Devin, wanted to be involved in the birth and was excited to be where the action was. We all hung out together, laughing and enjoying good food, as if it were just another day, visiting with friends.

When I had a contraction, I would lean on Devin and he would jokingly say in my ear, "Bring it around town, Mom! Bring it around town!" This is one of SpongeBob's silly sayings, from the television show. As I rocked my hips through the contraction, I laughed and smiled at him. After a few contractions, I went and ate some of my favorite chocolate. As I took a bite, I savored the delicious flavor in my mouth and was so thankful to be eating it. It tasted so good! I felt joyful and content with every bite.

As the night wore on, we watched the movie *Tenacious D.*, starring actor, Jack Black. I loved the satire of this film. I laughed *so* much during the movie. It made labor pleasurable, easy and fun. I *love* heavy metal music and it is part of who I am. Of course it should be part of my birth, since it brings me so much joy! Watching *Tenacious D* was a highlight of my self-designed experience.

I remember being told by my hospital-based midwife that my preferred style of music wouldn't be "conducive to birth." She told me to listen to nature sounds instead, like the sounds of whales or loons. I probably don't have to tell you that about an hour into listening to loon calls, I was ready to throw the CD player out the window. It wasn't something I enjoyed. *Fuck* relaxation! I want to enjoy and love what I listen to in life. Why should birth be any different?

Relaxation alone, as the main goal in labor, is simply not enough to focus on in preparing for birth. To be honest, it isn't even the direction one should be looking, if they want a positive experience in bringing their baby into this world. I feel this is where every other birthing method is *dead wrong* in its education of birth preparation. Telling a woman that *relaxation is the key to a natural birth* is misleading and setting a woman up for frustration and confusion–because forced relaxation during labor and birth isn't natural! Some women may relax *instinctually* during early labor, but not all women should do this. They should instead just do what their body is telling them to do, in complete partnership with their child.

I have learned through my own experiences and through supporting other women, that relaxation is *not* the main key to labor as previously thought. I do think that one can be relaxed and in an allowing state, if they are happy and *feeling good*; but to focus on relaxation, when it isn't natural to do so, doesn't allow her to do what she needs to do for her own unique, personal journey to birth.

As my labor progressed with Orion late into the evening, I told everyone to go to bed. I crawled into bed myself, and began thinking about how perfect the birth was going to be. I slept as much as I could between contractions. I would be gently awakened by the tightening and energy surging through my body. I would say over and over again in my head, "Yes! Yes!" I had a "Bring It!" attitude! I stayed in the most confident, powerful mindset that I could. I welcomed the contractions and whispered to

Orion that we were doing this together and that it would be so much fun. I let him know that we were partners and that I couldn't wait to hold him. I also told him to take his time, that we had all the time in the world.

I had read that clitoral stimulation during contractions could turn the strength of contractions into something extremely pleasurable. I was alone in the room and I hesitantly tried it during a contraction. It really worked!! Pleasure surged through my entire body in a way that I had never felt before! Now, this isn't something that I would have *ever* done if anyone else was there. This is why I share that an unassisted birth or laboring alone allows you to tap into a side of yourself that you couldn't with birth attendants, no matter how naturally-minded they are.

It was then that I realized the connection between sexuality and birth. I learned how good it could feel when you work with your instinctual ability to give yourself pleasure during labor. I knew that someday I would share this information with the world, with all of my inhibitions aside, so women could have a greater understanding of their power and potential.

After a while, I needed to get up and move! Changing positions in labor is something most women naturally want to do. It is all part of the process. Usually as the labor switches gears and goes to the next level of intensity, a woman has the urge to move around, or at least change positions, activity or scenery.

Joe heard me go into the bathroom and he came in to check on me, just as the sun was coming up. I hugged him and when I did, I had a strong, intense contraction. We rocked together until it was over. Then I told him that I had read that eye contact and kissing was helpful during hard labor. He smiled and with the next contraction he and I began kissing passionately and slowly.

Amazingly, it was as if we were both sharing the strength and powerful energy of the contraction. It was AMAZING. That kiss allowed me to share with him the power of labor and the experience in a way that is difficult to describe. It was if the energy was encircling us both in sensual connection. It was the first time that we understood and allowed the continuum of our love into physical form.

We gazed into each other's eyes and shared how much we loved one another. We rocked together as the sun came up and shared each and every contraction through eye contact and passionate, kissing.

An interesting observation that I made during hard labor, when Joe and I were kissing, was that you can't make out and not be relaxed and joyful! With every sexy kiss, I could feel my cervix opening wider and wider. It wasn't painful, it was *powerful*. Joe didn't tell me that, "I was doing great," like he'd repeated over and over again to me during my previous labors. This time he told me that I was sexy and hot and he shared "naughty" desires that he had for me.

This was very different than the culturally expected role of "support person" that he had been in the past. With Orion's birth, it was true and utter partnership. Through honoring our love and the sexual nature of our relationship, he thrust himself into another role, *entirely.* It was a role that felt much more natural and authentic. In being more truly who we were, I experienced a labor that was not only painless, but very pleasurable as well.

Hard labor was beautiful and I was thrilled that we made the conscious choice to be alone during that time. I was sharing the labor *with* him and he was taking on half of the work of letting go and allowing.

The most ideal support in labor isn't about the scripted words and back rubs. Sensually connecting is the most helpful and real. Experiencing labor like we did for Orion's birth, was the most romantic moment that we have ever had in our twenty years together, as a couple.

When you feel sexy during labor, you feel Goddess-like and full of self-confidence. One way a woman can help achieve this, is through buying a sexy, silky nighty to labor in. Wearing something that feels sexy to you will enable you to maintain your vision of birth being a continuum of your love and the fact that you are a sexual being. This will allow you to experience birth as sensual and highly pleasurable.

For my last, empowered birth, I shopped online and in lingerie stores. Trust me when I say that you DO get some funny looks, waddling into Victoria's Secret for "labor wear," when you are in your last trimester of pregnancy. I found the most beautiful, sexy night gown and luxurious robe that went along with it. When I got home, I put them on and felt like a total Goddess! "Now THIS is the way I want to birth!" I told myself. I also picked up some yummy smelling lotions and oils for the big day.

Feeling beautiful and sexy is an aspect of the birthing process that you never hear about, but it is so very important on many levels. When we feel confident in how we look, we feel confident in how we birth. Now saying this may make me an outcast in the naturally-minded birthing community, but I have found it to be very true with the women I work with, as a Doula.

There is a sort of spiritual snobbery proclaiming that looks shouldn't matter and that only "inner beauty" should matter. In my own experience, this isn't true or based in reality. It is an abstract ideal. It is denying, in a way, that we are both spiritual and physical beings. Why would we nurture one aspect of ourselves, and not another? Feeling beautiful is your right as a woman, and the way you look and feel, embarking on your labor, has a profound impact on the experience. Invest time into spiritual, mental *and* physical preparation, and you will have a balanced, pure focus heading into your birth.

I always buy my clients a sexy nightgown as a gift for labor, and they *love* it! The women that I work with often share that feeling goddess-like, allowed them to tap into the divine, confident energy within themselves. Wearing an old T-shirt just doesn't bring the same confidence. Feeling frumpy brings you down on the vibrational scale, and this is *not* the optimal place to be during such a sacred time in your life. Honoring yourself during this divine time of birth, and adorning your body is a personal sign of respect for oneself. This is something greatly lacking in today's understanding of the birth process! When you feel sensual fabrics on your skin during labor, it feels so good! It allows you to be in a state of "YES!" energy. This is exactly the space you want to be to birth joyfully. It is the same vibrational state you are in when conceiving and feeling your sexiest!

Having your dilation checked during pregnancy and in labor, does little to give any kind of accurate information about how long the labor will be. It is a medical measurement, but it is so flawed. Even some homebirth midwives still use this method of measuring a woman's progress, but it does carry some risks, both mentally and physically.

There is always a risk of infection every time anyone is reaching into your vagina, even with gloves on. There is also a risk of the person rupturing your membranes, and if this happens with a hospital birth, you have to deliver the baby within twenty-four hours, per hospital policy. This usually leads to intervention and medication, in order to ensure the birth happens within twenty-four hours of the membranes rupturing. The baby isn't really ready to be born, but because of liability and safety–in the eyes of the medical professionals–the birth is encouraged.

The second reason why checking dilation is flawed and dangerous, is that it tells you nothing about how much longer it will be until the birth, or how long labor is going to be. I have witnessed women going from two to ten centimeters, in two hours; and then on the other end of the spectrum, it takes some women days or weeks to dilate from two to ten centimeters.

If labor has been long and the woman is checked and finds out that she is only three centimeters dilated, the emotional disappointment may be enough to pull the rug right out from underneath her. If a woman has been in labor for two days, and then hears this information, she may feel such self-doubt that she decides not to go on. She does the flawed, medical-based math in her head, and then figures it will be *days* before she gives birth!

This is so unfortunate, because a woman can take a long time to dilate to two or three centimeters, only to open very quickly–in *minutes* sometimes– all the way to fully dilate! It can crush a woman emotionally, and throw her completely down the vibrational scale, to hear that all of her hard work is being perceived as "non-productive."

It is so important that the support people assure her that dilation *tells you nothing* as to how much longer labor will be and to maintain her positivity and joy surrounding the birth. Better yet, don't have dilation checked at all! There is nothing beneficial for the mother or baby in doing so.

I have seen a woman's birth team deflate with disappointment upon hearing that a woman is only two centimeters dilated, after they have been supporting her for many hours. Even if the support people never say a word about it, a woman can *feel* their disappointed and fearful energy. Do not underestimate this! A woman in labor has heightened senses and perception of even the most subtle change in the emotions of those around her.

A slight shift in energy is sometimes all it takes for a woman to lose her confidence. It is of vital importance to learn to trust birth yourself, and educate yourself about what is normal during labor, if you are going to be part of a woman's labor support team. Learn what is normal for a natural labor and birth. This way, you can always carry the energy of love and trust, and not only support her physically, but emotionally and energetically as well.

It is a personal choice as to whether to be checked or not, but you *always* have an option. It may never be presented to you as such; so always be sure to be assertive if you are told someone is going to check your dilation. I recommend that you confidently and kindly state that you choose not to be checked. This is an opportunity to be a voice for your baby.

8

HOT SHIFTS IN CONSCIOUSNESS

If dilation tells you nothing as to how long labor is going to be, how do we know how far along a woman is, in the labor process? The answer is simple – it is by observing her shifts in **consciousness**. By consciousness, I mean the laboring woman's awareness and understanding of her needs, behavior and attitudes.

When a woman is in early labor, she is pretty much herself. She will usually be excited, and if it is during the day, she likely feels like moving around. She may stop during contractions and rock back and forth, close her eyes, or gently moan through contractions; but as soon as they are finished, she continues on with whatever she was doing.

She can also easily carry on a conversation, and she stays focused and positive about the journey that lies ahead. This is a great time to go for a walk together, enjoy a nice dinner–abundant with her favorite foods, or watch a funny movie. It is a good idea to line these things up ahead of time, and plan together what you'll eat, watch and do. If labor begins in the middle of the night, sleep or rest would be the best option.

Early labor is usually the longest part of labor. It can be fun, playful and exciting! A woman in labor is aware of everything around her and her senses are heightened. Her clarity and focus are sharp. Love is the guiding energetic force during this time; and feeling like a goddess connected to the thousands of other women on Earth, who are laboring at the same exact time, is sublime.

As labor progresses to what our culture refers to as "hard labor," a woman usually shifts in consciousness, to a more inward focus. To someone observing her, she may not seem as connected to you, and this is good and normal. Nature has led her to focus now on her body and her baby. The outer world dims in comparison to what she is experiencing, and if asked a question, the woman will usually answer with the fewest words possible.

It can be hard for the woman's partner to feel this disconnect, if he is insecure or fearful. It is so important not to make it "about you" during this time, and allow her this shift in consciousness. I have witnessed nurses and doctors almost insisting that a woman focus on them, during this stage, and it is a kind of emotional and energetic torture of sorts. It is so disrespectful of the sacredness of this time in a woman's experience.

A woman needs quiet and the utmost respect, as the labor progresses. Dim lights and music that she loves are important to further encourage her to go inward, and tap into her inner strength and inner knowing that *all is well, perfect and as it should be.*

A woman is usually no longer hungry during this time, but she may get thirsty; so you can put some water, juice or her favorite beverage nearby, so she can easily reach it.

The energy of love and allowing is the predominant space that I hold for women in labor. Just smiling and being in the mindset of confidence and trust is so important. Loving the woman is so essential too!

Having love for whomever I am working with, as a Doula, has been one of my greatest assets to working with her. We all have the ability to love, but in our culture–even as birth workers– we are trained to keep it all business. We aren't encouraged to connect with the women whom we work with. Yes, we are told to be their "friends," but in such a sacred role of being part of their birth–well, how can love not come into the picture? How can love not be part of the experience? It is essential for the woman to be loved by those that surround her, during this time.

Loving and honoring *myself* while attending births, is something I value as well. Women energetically mirror those that walk with her on her journey. When we love ourselves, so do they. I wear beautiful clothes and get ready for the birth as if I am attending the most sacred of events. I would never think of showing up at a birth, only wearing sweat pants and a t-shirt. It simply isn't respectful to do so.

I always put aside a beautiful, silky shirt and comfortable, beautiful flowing pants to wear for the birth. I oftentimes put flowers in my hair from my garden too. I never wear strong scents, unless the woman wants me to. I know that with her heightened senses, certain smells can be overwhelming for a laboring woman.

I hold the space for all that she is and all that the experience will be for her. Honoring her from the inside out is very important. I treat the birth as the very sacred ceremony that it is.

There is a time between hard labor and pushing, when some women experience incredible emotional intensity. This sometimes manifests in fear, panic or pain. It is usually called "transition." Only a small percentage of women have a challenging transition and it usually only lasts about twenty minutes to an hour.

However, it is important to be aware that it is normal, and a sign that everything is progressing perfectly. Sometimes women go through self-doubt during this time. Sometimes they vomit, and sometimes they just burp a lot! It is a very powerful time, no matter how she experiences it.

It is the switching of gears, of sorts, and a shifting of energy. The contractions begin to feel expulsive at their peak, and this change can be intense and something to get used to. It is also a time when you realize that there is no turning back–your baby is coming! It is exciting, emotional and extremely powerful.

When I am with a woman who is experiencing a challenging transition, if she begins saying things like, "I can't do this anymore!", I smile knowing that she will begin pushing very soon. Self-doubt, for many women, is the indicator that she is shifting gears and going to the next phase–the actual birth itself.

I support the woman during this time in various ways, but verbally I share that self-doubt is good! It means she is surrendering. I encourage her to allow this intense energy to flow through her. I share that she is not alone and she is loved.

For most women, however, they never go through self-doubt or fear. They tap into the great energy and allow it to swirl around them. You can literally feel energy building, then exiting your body when you are opening fully, just before you begin pushing. It is incredible!

I remember squatting and leaning on the bed in front of me, while in labor with Orion. I felt like I was an energetic conductor and simply allowed the powerful energy to move through me. It was like conducting lightning, but much more pleasurable!

Instead of being hit with it and fighting it, you conduct it, by simply allowing it to flow through you. It felt indescribably good! By *allowing*, instead of resisting, you do not feel pain. You feel intense *connection* to all that is.

Most cultures in the world do not fear birth, nor do they experience pain during childbirth. No mammal on Earth does, either. It is our culture's belief in pain being part of the process that literally creates the experience of childbirth being painful and difficult. When you research other cultures and those in our society, who are having painless and joyful births, you will begin to recondition your mind. Then, your beliefs will change. This is essential to having the kind of birth that I am sharing about. You also need to have a sense of worthiness and know that you deserve a joyful, positive birth experience. This sometimes takes a great deal of inner-work, but it is the basis from which all else grows.

Sexy Birth

9

PUSH AND ALLOW

Have you ever heard the term, "Don't push the river, it flows by itself"? It is a great metaphor for the pushing phase of birth. Women have only been told to push their babies out in the last hundred years or so, because doctors thought that this part of labor was dangerous for the baby. At one time, doctors even told women to push at the beginning of labor! In the 1950's they changed that belief to only pushing once the woman was fully dilated.

The reality is that a woman never has to push, unless she feels an overwhelming need and desire to. In fact, if a woman was unconscious, her body would push her baby out just fine! Interestingly enough, it is actually dangerous for the baby, to force pushing. I feel that it is also cruel and controlling to scream, "Push! Push!" when a woman is trying to tap into her own *inner knowing* about what her body is telling her to do!

Your body will tell you when to push–Period. It may not be until the baby is crowning! I have seen babies be harmed during this phase, when the woman was told to push for too long. It depleted the baby and mother of much needed oxygen, and exhausted them both as well. Brain damage has been reported in babies whose mothers were told to push long and hard, before their bodies were ready to do so. Just because a woman is fully dilated, does not mean that she needs to start pushing! She should instead, do what feels best to her.

Sometimes a woman wants to sleep for a while, or sometimes she may want to move around or take a shower. In our culture, we make birthing much harder than it has to be! This is another reason why the idea of pain is so prevalent. Pushing, when your body isn't ready, really hurts! Pushing is supposed to feel good!

Pushing is a lot like having a bowel movement–which I know, isn't very sexy. It is natural, however, and very little effort is needed to accomplish this normal human function–when you don't have someone else controlling or managing it.

Can you imagine the damage that you would do to your insides, if you woke up and began pushing for hours before you really had to go? Imagine people screaming in your ears, "Keep going! Push!" Yes, eventually you would have a bowel movement, but so much wasted energy and damage to your body would occur, as a result of having someone else dictate and control the experience. When you have the freedom to find your own way, birth is easy, instinctual and joyful.

Birth is all about allowing, and realizing that you are capable of the intensity of all of the sensations of labor. Realize that the sensations of labor and birth aren't something happening to you, they *are* you! Nature has created the perfect, individualized birth that is designed specifically for you and your child.

Beginning a life in partnership with your baby is very important. It lays the foundation of a connected life together. Your baby is not scared or doubting during his birth, so why should you be? He trusts at a level that ensures his own well-being. If you aren't in vibrational alignment with that, you create risks for yourself and your baby that would never be present if you stayed in your natural state of joy and trust of the process.

Did you know that you will not tear if you allow birth to unfold in this way? Your vagina is meant to stretch amazingly well, if you allow it to do so at nature's rate, without forced pushing.

Tearing seems like a natural occurrence, but unless the baby is posterior or some other variation comes into play, tearing is extremely rare! I never tore with my eleven pound son and my ten pound daughter, because I allowed my body to guide me, without anyone dictating how I should be doing things. With my first birth, which was in a hospital with a midwife, I tore. This was because I had the typical cheering section on either side of me screaming, "You can do it! Push! Push!" They were also counting loudly and controlling what I did. I suppose they wanted to feel useful and their ego fed their management of my experience.

Pushing at home with my second child, I was pleasantly surprised with how easy it was. Dakota eased out of my body painlessly during this phase, and it actually felt *really* good, like a release–much like a bowel movement feels, but with heightened intensity and relief.

No matter where you choose to birth, if you are birthing with others present, be sure to let them know that you do not want the "cheering section" during pushing. Inform those attending that you prefer quiet during this time. Let them know that you also do not want time limits on pushing. Most hospitals have two hour time limits, in which to push, before they order a Cesarean or force intervention.

The time limits on pushing in a hospital are unfortunate, because the average pushing time for women, especially with first births, is anywhere between twenty minutes and six hours! This is all within the range of normal and to limit the time, for liabilities sake, isn't something that you should allow.

Remember, you are paying the doctors, nurses and midwives to *work for you*. You have options and choices and need to assert yourself to ensure that your choices are respected and honored. If you don't know your options, you don't have any. Ask your caregiver if they have a time limit on pushing, and if they do, find a new care provider!

10

HARD CORE RESPONSIBILITY

Rape and making love. Both are the same *physical* act, but they each create extremely different emotions and outcomes. One is painful and victimizing and damages women emotionally– possibly for the rest of their lives. One is a beautiful, loving, connected experience that forever enriches their lives, through creating children and strong emotional bonds. What does this have to do with birth?

I feel that we live in a victimizing culture. Things are improving, but for most people today, being raised in a victim mindset means that one never has to take real responsibility for their lives.

Our culture perpetuates women as victims, especially when it comes to birth. We are shown as weak individuals being tortured by our bodies and our babies, during the experience, that by nature, is meant to empower us.

We are so conditioned to be in this victim role, that most women unconsciously enter birth with this belief deeply ingrained in their minds. Women, in a sense, expect to be tortured–as if birth is something happening *to* them, instead of the reality of the experience: that labor and birth is an extension of who they are.

When we take full responsibility for our births, we never have to be victims who need to be rescued. We can be strong, capable, empowered women who will grow, as we are meant to, by stepping up and making choices, instead of letting someone else do that for us.

When we turn our responsibility and power over to others, those people have their own agenda. It is not necessarily in our best interest, it is in theirs; and it is usually steeped in fear and coming from a perspective of wanting to feed their own ego. When we don't take full responsibility for our births, we run the risk of a physically and emotionally damaging experience that we will carry with us forever.

Just because birth, as a physical act, may look the same from woman to woman, *it is not*. It can empower you, or leave you feeling as a victim. It is *your* choice and your responsibility to create the experience that you want, by making informed, educated choices.

Unfortunately in our culture, when someone has been victimized they often times feel justified in treating others the same way they have been treated. I have been part of births where even the female obstetrician keeps the woman in the role of being submissive and obedient. The woman complies, because this is the cultural dynamic they are so used to. They never think anything of it!

Or, victims blame others for their pain and suffering, refusing to take responsibility for themselves or the outcomes of their choices in childbirth. I am not necessarily blaming the victim here, because the truth is, most women do not even know there are choices! One thing that I always tell my students is, "If you don't know your options, you don't have any."

When a woman jumps on the treadmill of our culture's current birthing system, from the very beginning, she is given very little responsibility. She is trained from the first prenatal visit to let others care for her. Although this may feel comfortable and familiar to women, the birth that unfolds from this is disempowering and unfulfilling.

When we let others make our decisions and just mimic what others have done, we will also get their result–which is most commonly a negative experience and a disassociation from one's body and baby. The birth experience ends up being a reason to become a victim and perpetuates the myth of childbirth.

Women love to share their "war stories" when it comes to birth. It is as if it is a competition to see who suffered the most. It is a negative ritual which only cuts one another down, instead of lifting each other up, like we should be doing as sisters on this planet. When we are all connected and treat one another with reverence and respect, we will, in turn, be treated the same way. Karma rocks like that!

So the bottom line is that you can have a birth on a similar vibration as rape, or you can have a birth on the same vibration as making love. It is all your choice and your experience will be based on your personal choices on your journey. You can be a cork on the ocean, being thrown about by the waves, controlled by the current, or you can take the bow lines of your ship and sail in the direction that you want to go!

How your baby comes into this world sets the foundation for their entire life experience and the rest of yours. It is something to take very seriously, joyfully and confidently. It is during pregnancy that you prepare, create and ensure that you are not a victim. You are a powerful woman, taking the responsibility to self-design your birth and your life.

11

Your Seductive Setting

The environment in which you labor and birth, must be created from a place of awareness of what is needed, so one can birth in peace and joy. The environment is something you can create and control. It is a place in which you can unleash your creative expression! However you decide to set the stage, it will profoundly affect the birth experience. When you think of the environment in which you *conceived* the baby, you can see how an environment of romance is desirable to *birth* your baby.

Dim lights, candles, and your favorite music will help to keep you on a positive, joyful vibe. This is exactly what you want for birth! Can you imagine how different it would be to make love under florescent lights, with machines beeping, and the sound of strangers walking by and coming in and out of the room? If a hospital birth is what you truly desire, can you imagine how the fearful, sterile, white, cold environment of the hospital will feel, if you don't take the responsibility to change it?

A positive environment is easy to create if you are birthing at home. Birthing in a hospital takes a little bit more work to negotiate, but it can be done! As a doula, I have turned hundreds of hospital rooms into romantic, sensual, relaxing spaces. It just takes a bit of communication and planning.

If you are planning a hospital birth, visit the hospital ahead of time and see if there is anything in the labor room that makes you uncomfortable. For some women, it is the clock. Most women have no desire to know what time it is while they are laboring. If this is the case, I make note of it and I am sure to cover the clock when we get there. The table of shiny instruments and the biohazard bucket are also uncomfortable and environmentally negative.

As a doula, I often visit the hospital with my clients, and I get a good feel for what the expectant Mom feels good or bad about, in the birthing room. Later on, when we are there and she is actually in labor, I create the space that she wants–from hanging fabrics, to putting candles around the room, to bringing in fresh flowers and aspects of nature. I know how truly important the environment is that a woman births in, and I take this aspect of my role very seriously. I want my clients to birth in pure peace and joy.

Music or funny, enjoyable DVD's are *essential,* since there are so many loud, negative sounds, which are part of the hospital environment. You can easily drown out the sounds of nurses at the nurse station, or the intercom alerting that there is a "Code Red in room 196." All of these environmental distractions affect the birth in a negative way. So to ensure a good experience, one where you won't get knocked off your high vibe, think of ways to make the room as much like home as possible. This can be accomplished by covering and masking the hospital's scary and intimidating sights and sounds.

When a primitive woman is in the jungle birthing, and feels a threat of an animal nearby, her labor stops. Once she feels safe again, the labor will get back into its natural rhythm and resume, as it was. This is a protective mechanism seen in all mammals.

The same is true for birthing women everywhere. When a woman first arrives at the hospital, it is really common for the labor pattern that she had going at home, to slow down, or even stop. This is normal and it is what is supposed to happen! Unfortunately, the medical perspective doesn't recognize that it is a natural response to fear in labor, and they usually view it as a problem. They will often scare the woman into accepting drugs to "get the labor going again."

This is unnecessary and almost always causes the cycle of intervention to begin. All the woman usually needs is to get settled in, and release the initial fear and anxiety associated with the trip and arrival. Those who love the laboring woman can create a supportive, joyful environment, and her labor will usually pick up where it left off at home.

If you are birthing at home, whether with midwives or unassisted, creating your nest can be so much fun! I created a very beautiful space in our bedroom, and covered cluttered storage shelves with pink sheets. I put fresh flowers *everywhere,* when I knew that labor was getting close. I also hung inspiring quotes all over the room–even on the ceiling. Vanilla scented candles and photos of friends and family decorated the tables, and my birth kit was ready to go, neatly, next to the bed. I made sure the space was clean and organized, because this puts me in an allowing, joyful state of mind.

I also created a birth CD, with all of my favorite music. This was exactly what I needed to be my most authentic self; and it was the missing piece from my other three labors, when I had chosen what I was "supposed" to be listening to for relaxation–according to other birth professionals. I am grateful that I learned that through being *authentically yourself* in labor and birth, it creates the most natural, joyful and pleasurable experience!

During hard labor and pushing, I listened to *Rage Against the Machine, Metallica* and other powerful, rhythmically aggressive bands. I moved my head up and down to the grinding rhythms during contractions. Most birth professionals would have scoffed at the music that I chose, because they may not view heavy metal music as being "conducive to birth."

I love to share about this because it is never about the *music itself*. It is about how the music makes the woman *feel*. Heavy metal music is an expression of who I am, and listening to it in labor made me feel powerful and confident. You need to choose music that makes you feel alive, powerful and connected to who you are!

During my labor with Orion, after Joe and I had romantically connected in the bathroom, I filled up the bathtub and soaked, while labor reached its peak of intensity. As my cervix opened fully, I said over and over again out loud, "I can do this! I can do this!" After a while, I knew it was time to push. I got out of the tub and got ready for the birth of my son. I slipped on my sexy, lacy nighty, which made me feel like a gorgeous, sexy birthing goddess! I lit the candles myself, between my intensely powerful contractions. I could feel him moving down, and I wanted his birth to be in pure love and joy.

Allowing the process to unfold, without fear or resistance, was essential in beginning a life in partnership with my son. Orion was already in this natural state of non-resistance and allowing. It was *I* who had to consciously ensure that I stayed there, without becoming fearful. Fear causes pain and complications in birth.

It is through resisting that the entire cultural paradigm of birth is based! It is only through fear and resistance that birth is difficult, complicated and painful. I was in complete trust and welcomed the sensations; and in doing so, the birth of my son was painless, and as it should be, by the laws of nature.

As I turned up my music, my whole body surrendered to the process; and within a couple of pushes, I was ready for my mother to come in and catch him. She came in and told me later that she was stunned that I was already pushing. It was perfect, and better than I had even envisioned. I knew it would be. After all, I created and designed the entire experience myself. My mother was forever changed after seeing birth as it was meant to be.

12

SEXY THOUGHTS = SEXY EXPERIENCE

When I was pregnant with Orion, I had learned about my power to create whatever I wanted in life, including the perfect, painless, joyful birth that I had. It was better than I ever dreamed it could be. I learned that my thoughts become my reality and that what I focus on most, would manifest in my life.

I realized how powerful my thoughts were from my last two birth experiences. They were extremely contrasting in every way. I am very grateful for them both, because I learned a great deal to be able to help others create the births that they want. The Universe doesn't hear that you *don't* want something. It only hears your dominant vibration and what you are focused on most.

Regarding Ivy's birth, I think it is important to mention that I didn't just have a *small* fear of a posterior labor and birth. I had a fearful *obsession*. I don't want you to think that fears in birth will automatically bring your fear into reality. Some fear is normal and healthy. It is when fears become habitual and destructive that they become an obstacle to our well-being.

If you do have a particular fear surrounding birth, it is often times because you are on a low vibration emotionally, to begin with. There is a scale of emotions that we all have. Fear is on the low end of it. When you are aware that you are the creator of your experience and your life, you can take responsibility to move yourself up the vibrational scale to help you create the life you want.

It can be difficult at first, but once you see how powerful your thoughts are and how powerful YOU are, you will begin to see how important it is to allow your fears to flow through you. Feel them, observe them without judgment, and then move on and up the emotional scale, to a better feeling place.

Even though there are countless shades of emotions that continuously ebb and flow, Abraham-Hicks', in their book "Ask and it is Given," shares their *Emotional Guidance Scale* so you can better see how you can climb up to a better feeling place. When you use this same scale about your feelings surrounding birth, you can use it as a tool.

1 . Joy/Appreciation/Empowered /Love
2 . Passion
3 . Enthusiasm/Eagerness/Happiness
4 . Positive Expectation/Belief
5 . Optimism
6 . Hopefulness
7 . Contentment
8 . Boredom
9 . Pessimism
10. Frustration/Irritation/Impatience

11. Overwhelment
12. Disappointment
13. Doubt
14. Worry
15. Blame
16. Discouragement
17. Anger
18. Revenge
19. Hatred/Rage
20. Jealousy
21. Insecurity/Guilt/Unworthiness
22. Fear/Grief/Depression/Despair

If you are in a lower vibration emotion, you can move up this scale; but you can't just jump from depression to Joy *instantly*. You have to move through the other emotions first. Moving from fear, to anger, to hope, to joy is much easier to do than to move from fear or depression, straight to Joy.

Expressing emotions, even negative emotion, is normal and natural. It is through being aware that your feelings and thoughts create your reality, that you can take the power into your own hands and change things for the better! When you can learn to be grateful for your experiences, even negative ones, you can change the painful memories of your past, into grateful moments of personal growth in the present.

I have learned so much from looking back on my birth with Ivy. Before I realized that I create my own experiences in life, I was disempowered. I now see that by focusing on what I *didn't* want during my labor and birth with Ivy, I created exactly that!

Through fear, I designed her birth from a very low place on the emotional scale. Through "preventative" action, I put so much energy on specifically what I didn't want, that the only thing the Universe heard was, "Posterior birth!" How interesting that I was *that* powerful! Instead of realizing it, I was in a fearful mindset and created the experience from that space.

Depending on where you are on the scale, you will attract people and circumstances that resonate with the same scale as your most habitual emotion. For instance, if you are consistently feeling powerless, you are bound to attract negative people and situations that keep you trapped in the state of powerlessness.

On the other hand, if your dominant emotion is that of love and gratitude, you are more likely to encounter positive situations that give you the same feelings. *We create our lives from the inside out, not the outside in.*

Choose Better Feeling Thoughts About Birth!

So in order to attract what you want for your birth, you need to shift your emotions from those lower on the scale, to those higher on the scale, by consciously focusing your thoughts, from negative to more positive. You can do this by deliberately choosing better feeling thoughts, each time you feel fearful about giving birth, until you move from a lower emotional state, to a higher one. When you learn how to do this, you will be able to climb out of states of fear or despair into optimism, enthusiasm, or even joy!

The more you do this, the easier it gets. When you see how important it is to own your emotions, you can create the reality you want for yourself. At first, you have to consciously choose to do this; but after a while, doing what you need in order to feel good becomes second nature. **The best thing you can do to ensure a**

joyful birth outcome, is to feel good now. It is your only job.

One way to help yourself shift thoughts and feelings is to do something that brings you joy. You might bake a cake, watch your favorite funny movie or call a friend. When I am feeling low on the vibrational scale, listening to music that I love always helps raise my vibe! I also love watching empowering births online or reading inspirational birth stories. The point is that it is *your* responsibility to shift how you are feeling–instead of feeling like a victim. Take the power into your own hands and do something to change how you feel, because how you feel is the space from which you are creating your outer life.

Joy is our most natural state, so in order to have a natural joyful birth, helping yourself feel more joy, would be the best thing you could do to bring that about! You can't wait for others to do it for you. Be empowered! Step up and start today! You will be amazed at how you can change your life by changing your thoughts.

Realizing your ability to direct your thoughts and feel better, no matter what happens, leads to accessing your full power to manifest what you truly desire in life. This little shift in thinking is powerful and it will change your life. By realizing your power now, you can drop negative thinking and victimization before your child even enters the world! What an amazing model you will be for your child, by taking full responsibility for your life and creating exactly what you want. You will be giving them a whole, powerful parent.

By having an optimistic attitude about labor and birth and by focusing on a joyful, healthy experience, you attract a joyful, healthy birth! While having a cynical, fearful attitude, you attract a negative birth experience. Change your thoughts and change your reality! **Having a *Sexy Birth* is really that simple!**

13

THE GODDESS SHOWER

We live in a society that is very focused on material things. This is why the Baby Shower is the predominant pre-baby celebration. It is all about the gifts; and although this is helpful for new parents starting out, it has nothing to do with the birth itself or honoring the woman who is transitioning to motherhood.

Something that is much deeper and more meaningful is what I call a *Goddess Shower*. This is an alternative to a baby shower, and is inspired by the traditional Native American blessing way ceremony.

A Goddess Shower is a celebration to show the mother-to-be how adored, supported and loved she is, in preparation for birth. It is a very meaningful and memorable time, in which a woman comes together with her friends and family, to celebrate birth as a poignant and powerful rite of passage.

I have been hosting and leading birth celebrations for many years, and with each and every one of them, I am brought to a higher level of understanding of the importance of such a gathering.

I recently gave my sister-in-law, Allie, a Goddess Shower, and I am happy to share how I led the ceremony, to celebrate her as a woman and as a soon-to-be mother.

Before Allie's Goddess Shower began, I arranged the chairs and pillows into a circle. I decorated the chair for Allie with fresh flowers. I then sprinkled rose pedals all over the center of the circle and put a very short table in the center of the petals. I used some pretty fabric to cover the table and then added more fresh flowers, that I knew were Allie's favorites. Lastly, I put some tea light candles on top of the table.

Before Allie arrived, I cued up her favorite music and prepared her favorite foods to serve. I chose to serve decadent desserts that she desired, since it was an afternoon event.

A Goddess Shower is unlike a baby shower in many ways. It isn't a surprise for the mother-to-be, and in fact, she takes a large role in planning her own celebration! I worked closely with Allie to create a powerful experience, designed especially for her. I feel that the aspect of co-creation is so important for her to come away from the event, feeling deeply supported and moved.

In the invitation to the Allie's Goddess Shower, I asked that everyone bring a bead or charm to be strung on a necklace, for Allie to wear during her labor. I explained that in doing so, she carries a piece of all of us to her birth, that she can draw strength from when she needs it the most. Whether the bead or charm was old or new, I asked that it contain a special meaning about why they chose it, that each person can share at the celebration.

I also asked that if people wished to bring a gift, that it be something special to pamper Allie.

Before Allie's Goddess Shower began, I lit the candles in the center of the circle and several around the room, to create a soft, feminine ambiance. I had a foot bath waiting for her when she arrived, with her favorite scents and fresh flowers floating in it.

I had music of her choice playing, as well. The focus of Allie's shower was very feminine and sexy. I had pink fabrics and boas tied on chairs, and flowers and sensual smelling candles in abundance, all over the room. I wanted Allie and her guests to be awed when they entered the room. We had sexy foods, like strawberries dipped in chocolate and pink raspberry ginger ale, served in champagne glasses. I wanted everything to honor Allie's divine femininity.

When Allie and her guests arrived, everyone sat in the circle. My brother and Allie's mom were also present and I asked them to sit on either side of her. I'd made an elegant crown of flowers, which I gave to her mother, to place on Allie's head. I sat across from them in the circle.

I could see her awe and excitement, when she first took a seat in the comfortable rocking chair that I'd decorated with flowers. The energy in the room was exciting and powerful. My brother, being the only man attending, could see and feel how incredible it was that we were celebrating Allie's womanhood. He also looked at her with reverence as she sat, looking like a Goddess, with all of us there to honor her in every way.

Once everyone was seated, I said that as a culture, we do not come together in such a way to honor a mother-to-be. It is such an essential ceremony, important to emotional birth preparation. This tribal and family support is the missing link in our culture, when it comes to birth and motherhood preparation.

Before we began, I asked that no one share any horror stories of labor or birth, and that we only speak joyfully and positively of what lies ahead for Allie. I shared that this was a divine support circle of love, one that they were all specially chosen to be part of. I added that such an event is unlike anything most women have ever seen before, and that being chosen as a guest was an honor. I looked into Allie's eyes and let her know how grateful I was to be there to lead this powerful gathering. It was at this time that I could see tears welling up in her eyes. Everyone attending knew how powerful the shower would be, and the energy shifted to a level of quiet reverence. The Goddess Shower had begun.

I began the shower by asking that we go around, one by one, and share how we knew Allie and what endeared us to her. This was a time of tears and laughter, and everyone had an opportunity to connect with Allie, individually. It was especially powerful to hear her mother and her husband share. It is with this type of deliberate, organized support that a woman gains insight as to how loved and cherished she truly is. It is such a gift for her to hear how really loved and adored she is. It also brings the couple to a place of remembering what really matters, in the midst of everything else they are focused on in preparing for the birth of their baby.

After everyone shared how they met Allie and what endeared them to her, it was time to make her Goddess necklace. I put all of the beads on a beautiful tray, along with some hemp twine and spacer beads, which were put on the necklace, in between the individual beads and charms that the guests brought.

We began creating the necklace, by each of us sharing why we chose the bead or charm for Allie. Tears were shared and Allie expressed gratitude, as the necklace was created. As I tied it around her neck, I reminded her to bring it with her to the hospital, and to keep it in a place where she can see it throughout the labor and birth. I told her that it can be used as a tool to draw strength from, when she needs it the most, and that we would all be with her, symbolically, during labor and birth.

I remember sharing with Allie that even though not everyone who was there at the shower, would be at the birth physically, that we would all be there energetically for her, and that she is never alone. I told her that every hour that she is in labor, 16,000 women are giving birth worldwide, right along with her, and she can tap into that great, collective power. I told the guests that Allie was part of the great circle of life and love, and birth was a time to feel connected to every living thing on the planet. I shared that we are all One and that we are helping her through her incredible rite of passage to motherhood. The guests were moved by my words, and in that moment, we all felt connected on a deeper level.

After creating Allie's necklace, we broke from the circle for some sexy refreshments! I changed the music to something more upbeat, and I walked around and played hostess to ensure that everyone had a beverage and some decadent food. I offered Henna tattoos for those who wanted them. Allie also opened her pampering gifts and everyone enjoyed seeing her receive such fabulous, sexy items!

After about an hour of mingling and activities, I asked if everyone could return to the circle to close the ceremony. I asked that we all share a wish, hope or blessing for Allie's labor and birth. One by one, guests shared their loving well-wishes and wisdom, as a final gift for my sister-in-law. It was a very special ending to such a powerfully transformative ceremony. My brother was very moved by the love expressed for his wife. Allie's mother cried as she bore witness to her daughter's being treated and honored like a Goddess.

As each woman shared her wish for Allie, she lit a candle that was in the center of the circle. By the end of the shower, all of the candles were lit. I then shared that Allie could take the candles home and light them when she goes into labor. At that time, they will serve to bring our wishes into her reality.

Moving away from the materialistic focus of our culture, and shifting to a more heart-based, connecting ceremony, we give a woman such an incredible gift that she will carry with her for the rest of her life.

The Goddess Shower is something every woman deserves, at some point during her final weeks of pregnancy. It is something that I hope more and more women give their sisters, friends and loved ones, who are about to bring a baby into this world. It serves as a ritual, honoring the transformation of the woman, as she steps into life as a mother. It gives the woman the gift of the love and the focus being only on her, because once the baby is born, the focus shifts to the baby itself. It also serves as a healing and as a powerful way for those who love the woman, to connect with her in a way they never have before. In the decade that I have been leading Goddess Showers, I have observed that they are just as transformative to the guests, as they are to the mother-to-be.

Sexy Birth

Afterglow

Birth is something that women in our culture are finally taking back! We are the creators, nurturers and forces of love and light that cannot be dimmed, unless we allow others to manage and control our birthing experience. When we take full responsibility for how our babies enter this world, we have the power to change humanity for the better.

Times are changing. A new era of empowered, authentic women are coming forth to bring about change. YOU are part of this ever-widening circle of women. Being authentically who you are is profoundly sexy! When we honor our authenticity and take the responsibility for our thoughts, we can create the most, joyful, natural and healthy birth experience possible. When you meet your own needs and desires, all who come into contact with you will benefit.

It is through meeting our own authentic needs, that we model this example to our children. They learn from how we are in this world. When we love ourselves, our children love themselves. We begin this self-love through how we bring forth life. You are deserving of a Sexy Birth! Welcome to the beginning of your journey!

Acknowledgments and Thanks

I have been a doula and childbirth educator for ten years now. Through great inspiration and gratitude, I bring the last decade of my work to a book, which will hopefully impact lives and help shift the way our culture views birth and parenting. I couldn't have done this alone. I have enormous gratitude for the many people in my life that helped make this book possible.

Thank you to my husband and best friend, Joey, for encouraging and supporting me, in everything I do in life. I love you more than words can say. If it wasn't for your unconditional love, I wouldn't be who I am today. Thank you to my mother, Darlene, for always being there to listen to my ideas and tell me that I can have, do and be whatever I want to, in life.

Thanks to my children, Devin, Dakota (Tiff), Ivy and Orion, for allowing me to share the stories of their births with the world. I am so grateful to be your Mom. I love you all so much!

Thank you to my dearest friends, Liza, Rachel, Josha, Caitlin, Maree, Kelley, Christina and Kim. Your love and support mean the world to me!

Thank you to my amazing editor, Lynda Miles, for her ability to communicate clearly and with love. Thank you to my web designer and friend, Ted Olson, for his honest opinions and motivation. Thank you to Jay Philbrick for the incredible co-creation of the cover and back photos. Thank you to Tsiyon and Ian for the professionalism and love that shined through in the photos, just weeks before the birth of their son, Elijah. Thank you to Rileigh, my mother's helper, for being such an incredible role model for my children!

Thank you to my many students and Doula clients, who have allowed me the honor of being part of the experience of their children's births. It is through a decade of supporting couples and attending births, that I have learned the most about the power of a confident, sexy woman!

Thank you to the birth advocates and pioneers who have inspired me in my work: Ina May Gaskin, Suzanne Arms, Ricki Lake, Abby Epstein, Henci Goer and Christiane Northrup.

Last but not least, thank you to my growing community of online friends. I have been supported and blessed with friends from all over the world. They have affected my life in profoundly positive ways and for that, I am eternally grateful.

Printed in Great Britain
by Amazon

79339221R00102